FREE RESOURCES

Thank you for taking the time to read my book.
To help you on your weightless journey, I have included
2 discounts for Amazon Customers.

COUPON CODE HEALTH24
10% Off any Weight Loss Plan at
DrLoriMahler.com

COUPON CODE AZ12
New Client Virtual Consultation
45 Minute
Includes Nutrition Assessment

Email DrLoriMahler@gmail.com with Codes

I

Dr. Lori Mahler

SECRETS TO SUSTAINABLE WEIGHT LOSS

A Naturopathic Approach to Conquer Weight Loss, Break Sugar Addiction and Balance Hormones

By

Lori Mahler

Table of Contents

Introduction

In the US, it has been reported that forty-five million people try to lose weight each year and spend 33 billion dollars on weight loss programs and products. When it comes to losing weight, there are many unanswered questions and controversies about how to lose and maintain weight for life. Although many programs are on the market, very few teach us how to embrace maintenance in a way that does not make us feel like we are missing the good things in life. The truth is that there will never be a one-size-fits-all program because each of us has different imbalances in the body that are contributing to our weight struggles.

As you read the information in this book, I want to encourage you to set aside everything you think you know about how to lose weight and be open to a shift in your thinking. Weight loss is not just about calories in calories out, especially as we age, if you continue to struggle with the same obstacles on your weight-loss journey it is important to understand that excess fat is stored as a result of what is happening on the inside of your body.

Whether you have 10 or 100 pounds of weight to lose, it can make everyday life feel much more difficult. Excess weight impacts our lives in diverse ways. For many of us, it negatively affects our confidence, self-esteem, and body image. For others, it profoundly affects social interactions, relationships, and how we present ourselves to the world. When we do not feel comfortable in our bodies it is hard to show our true selves. There are also physical symptoms that come as a package deal with excess weight such as bloating, sugar cravings, brain fog, fatigue, and knee pain.

The content in this book will provide you with clear direction, next steps, and strategies to give you a roadmap to reach and maintain your weight loss goals. I will help you dig deep to determine "why" and "what" the potential barriers are making it difficult for you to lose weight and how to apply a naturopathic and integrated approach.

To those feeling hopeless in their weight loss journey and believing that medications, like Ozempic, are the only way forward. I want you to know that you are not alone, and there is still hope. Your body is not broken, and quick fixes or temporary solutions do not define you. Real, sustainable, transformation is possible- through nourishment, movement, mindset shifts, and self-compassion. It's not about perfection, but about reconnecting with your body, healing is your own pace and finding balance in a way that honors your unique needs. You are capable of far more than you realize, and the power to change lies within you. This journey won't be easy, but it will be worth it- and you're worth it

If you enjoy my book, please take a moment to leave a review on Amazon. This allows me the opportunity to help other customers like you feel confident that there is hope that they can reach their health goals too. Sharing your positive experience will be appreciated!

CHAPTER 1:
The Science of Weight Loss

Losing weight is a widespread problem these days and both men and women struggle with it at various times throughout our life. We battle with the scale, what to eat, calorie restriction, and belly fat. For women, we watch our husbands lose weight overnight. Men tend to lose weight quickly because they have more muscle mass but struggle to maintain it. When we ask for guidance on weight loss from our doctor, the typical answer is to eat less and move more. Unfortunately, it is not always that simple. Negative eating patterns tend to start in childhood and continue throughout our high school years. Peer pressure, body image concerns, self-esteem issues, and trying to "fit in" can lead to an unhealthy relationship with food. When we have excess weight on our body, it makes life feel much more difficult.

If you are reading this book, then you either have been struggling or are currently trying to figure out why the scale is not moving. If you feel you are doing all the right things, avoiding temptations, eating healthily, and exercising but the weight does not budge, it can make you feel trapped in your own body. I understand exactly how you are feeling. At the age of thirty-two, I had reached my highest weight of 220 and I was experiencing symptoms that scared me; (sugar addiction, brain fog, rashes, debilitating anxiety, and pains in my abdomen. A doctor's appointment confirmed that I had high blood pressure, cholesterol, lupus, and pre-diabetes. I knew it was a consequence of the excess weight I was carrying. My doctor told me to lose weight, but he had no answers as to what I was to do other than to cut calories and exercise. I knew that did not work because I had already tried that and every diet program on the market. Nothing felt sustainable. He offered me a lengthy list of medications for all my health issues with an even longer list of side effects. I declined all the medications and at that moment, I knew I was on my own for the health journey that lay ahead of me.

That day, I left the doctor's office and began researching the one thing that I had not tried to lose weight. I went to five supermarkets and health food stores to look at the product labels of all the food I had eaten for the last few years. I started listing the products, the ingredients, and the so-called "healthy foods" that claimed to have zero sugar, low fat, or low carb. I came to realize all the junk that I had put in my body, food starches, fake sugars, artificial dyes, and chemicals. I could not understand why the FDA was allowing the manufacturers to put toxic chemicals into the products and was shocked to discover all the names that I could not pronounce on the product labeling. I researched the weight loss programs that I had once tried and failed at along with the 'weight loss foods" from Jenny Craig and Nutrisystem I realized that I had found the "root cause" of my weight issues. Throughout my research, I discovered that manufacturers used ingredients in their products.to help their products remain shelf stable.

I learned that they add chemicals to make their products look pretty (artificial dyes), starches and stabilizers, to thicken the products, and hundreds of other chemicals. I discovered over sixty chemical names for sugar that manufacturers disguise in the ingredient labels. Manufacturers do not make their products to help us achieve optimum health. Manufacturers can add what they want to their product labeling -and make false claims with little consequence from the FDA.

I decided to develop my nutritional plan based on what I was learning. I replaced all the processed foods with minimally processed or whole foods. I lost about two pounds every week for the first 3 months. I immersed myself in my education and could not believe how my body was changing. I felt great and my anxiety was almost non-existent. I continued steadily losing until I reached 180 pounds- and then my weight loss stalled again. This time I plateaued for 3 months even though I had eliminated all the processed foods and exercised regularly. I started to experiment with the amounts of proteins I was eating and religiously tracked my calories. I had been doing cardio and began incorporating more weights. That pushed me right through the plateau and I was back to losing 2-3 pounds a week. When I reached a scale weight of 160, my weight loss stopped again. I tried to make more adjustments, but nothing worked. At that time, I began my education at the School for Naturopathic Medicine, and I began to realize that my weight was not moving due to things going on internally in my body. Hormone issues, gut issues, and sluggish metabolism.

The key takeaway from my experience is that healthy eating, eating low carb and exercising can only take you so far if the body is out of balance. I felt excited but disappointed because I realized I needed to dig in and continue learning and applying the knowledge to reach my weight loss goal. I kept moving forward and began the healing process which consisted of natural medicine and herbs to address my body systems that needed support. At that point, I began my education on holistic nutrition and realized that not only is whole food nutrition and "real food" all that we should be eating but that "food is medicine" to our bodies if it is in its whole natural state. I reached my weight of 139 and have maintained it for 17 years. Now, as a naturopathic doctor and nutritional therapist, I am a firm believer that each of us has a calling. My goal is to empower you with knowledge, tools, and insight to help you reach your weight loss goals.

What is the Difference Between a Naturopathic Doctor vs a Conventional Medicine Doctor

As a naturopathic doctor, I address the same problems that medical doctors see every day in their offices. However, instead of treating a patient with medications that suppress symptoms, I work to find out what is causing undesirable conditions. Having a good understanding of your specific symptoms and body/organ/gland conditions, much can be learned about how your body expresses nutritional deficiencies the need to detoxify, weakened organ/glands emotional issues, and resistant weight loss. If you have a history of weight loss issues, it is safe to assume that your answer is not just about nutrition and exercise.

Finding the root cause of health conditions is an important aspect of natural health. Weight loss is no different. There are root causes to "why" your body is struggling to release weight. It could be one or more root causes. The end goal is to repair, heal, and support the body systems that are out of balance to reset the body.

In this subchapter, we will begin to delve into the science behind weight loss and help you identify the common root causes of your weight issues. As we age our metabolism does slow down, making it more challenging to shed excess pounds. However, learning more about the science behind your weight loss can empower you to make informed decisions and achieve your goals.

The Science Behind Weight Loss

Most nutritional gurus will tell you that the key to weight loss is to "eat less move more." This works for a while but your body will demand the right fuel to release weight. This is why people struggle to lose the last 10 to 15 pounds- they are not eating enough quality fuel. Many people who try to lose weight simply feel confused as to what and who to believe about weight loss. My answer to this is that a one-size-fits-all solution does not exist. Understanding your body, the imbalances, and applying the corrections that you need to make is the answer. I know this to be true based on my own experiences, research, and what I have seen with my clients for the past 13 years.

It is important to understand what fat is. Fat is stored tissue in the body, not energy. So, what tells your body to store fat? It is the hormone signal, the chemical signal, and the inflammatory signals that your body gets from the food you eat. It is typically not a calorie issue. When we eat fat, protein, or carbs, they each travel down a specific metabolic pathway in the body. The type of foods you eat plays a significant role in whether your body easily stores fat. Foods high in refined sugars and processed carbohydrates can lead to glucose spikes which is the recipe for excess fat storage around the belly, thighs, and hips. Whole food nutrition, achieving holistic balance internally, and learning to "listen" to your body are the "secret sauces" to achieving lifelong weight management.

Defining Processed Foods

When new clients come to me, they think they are eating healthily. They feel confused and right because in their mind they are doing what they are supposed to do to lose weight. It is important to have a good understanding of what processed foods are and what the typical consequences will be due to excess weight on the body.

Processed foods encompass a wide range of products that have undergone various methods of alteration from their original state. This includes anything from minimally processed items, such as pre-washed salads and frozen fruits, to heavily processed goods like sugary cereals, snack cakes, and instant noodles. The key distinction lies in the extent of processing and the types of ingredients used. While processed foods can be nutritious and convenient, others may contain elevated levels of sugars, unhealthy fats, and additives that can negatively affect health.

The best approach when using processed foods is to purchase from supermarkets such as Whole Foods, Trader Joe's, or high-end health food stores that offer products with minimally processed ingredients. Eating healthily is indeed expensive but when the health goal is to prevent disease and live a happy healthy and medicine-free life, then looking at expensive grocery bills each month is a worthwhile investment in your future. Another way to look at costly food purchases is to understand that you will either be paying more now for healthy food or later down the road for hospital bills due to disease in the body. Learn to be a label detective. Make the time to investigate and know what you are putting into your body.

Processed foods often contain a variety of additives and preservatives designed to enhance flavor, improve texture, and prolong shelf life. While these ingredients may serve practical purposes in manufacturing and distribution, and can have significant implications for health, particularly for women and their children. Understanding these additives is crucial for making informed dietary choices that prioritize well-being, especially in a landscape where processed food consumption is rising, and obesity rates are climbing. One of the most prevalent types of additives found in processed foods is artificial flavorings. These compounds mimic natural flavors to create an appealing taste profile without using real ingredients. For example, synthetic flavorings are derived from a wide range of sources, including chemicals not originally intended for consumption. While they can make foods more palatable, there are concerns that these artificial flavors may trigger allergic reactions or sensitivities-especially in children. whose developing bodies are more vulnerable. Additionally, repeated exposure to these flavors could lead to a preference for sweet or highly processed foods, (sugar addiction) further contributing to unhealthy eating habits.

Preservatives are another common category of additives, used primarily to inhibit spoilage and extend the shelf life of products. Preservatives, like salt and vinegar, are natural and have been used for centuries, many modern preservatives, such as BHA, BHT, and sodium nitrite, have raised health concerns. Research has suggested links between certain preservatives and health issues, including hyperactivity in children and potential carcinogenic effects. For women, particularly those who are pregnant or breastfeeding, the intake of these substances warrants careful consideration, as they may impact fetal development or affect nursing infants.

Coloring agents, both natural and artificial, are also frequently added to processed foods to make them visually appealing. Brightly colored snacks and beverages often attract children, masking the fact that these foods may lack essential nutrients. Artificial colorings have been associated with hyperactivity and behavioral issues in children. Parents need to read labels carefully and understand what these additives are, as they can influence not only taste but also overall health and well-being. Find a nutritionist in your area who specializes in children's meals and snacks to find the best healthy swaps and nutritionally balanced minimally processed foods that you can. While additives and preservatives can enhance the appeal and longevity of processed foods, their potential health implications should not be overlooked. Everyone should be aware of the common additives present in many of the foods that are the catalysts in developing weight issues, obesity, and diabetes. By prioritizing whole, minimally processed foods and being vigilant about ingredient lists, you can make healthier choices that contribute to better health outcomes. Understanding these hidden ingredients is a vital step in combating the rising obesity epidemic and achieving lifelong weight management.

High-Calorie Density Foods- Low Nutritional Value

One of the primary concerns regarding processed foods is their high-calorie density combined with low nutritional value. Most processed foods are made to be palatable and addictive, often containing excessive sugars, unhealthy fats, and sodium. This combination makes it easy to consume enormous quantities without feeling full, leading to overeating, and starting the process of hormone imbalance in the body. Sugar addiction and sugar cravings are typically the first signs that the body is becoming addicted to the 'sugars or chemical components in the food.

When we ingest food with no nutrient value, the body does not" register" or "understand" that it is being fed. This is why we can eat large volumes of processed food in one sitting and never feel full. Food is information, (code) to the body. You are giving it instructions on what to do. The body cannot extract anything other than chemicals and preservatives from manufactured processed food so its response will be to send the body down the path to disease, whereas whole food nutrients and low-calorie high-density food send us down the road to health and vitality within the body.

The marketing strategies employed by big food companies often glamorize processed foods, making them appeal to consumers of all ages. Colorful packaging, catchy slogans, and endorsements by popular figures create an illusion of health and desirability, particularly for children who are impressionable and easily influenced by advertisements. These marketing tactics skew perceptions of what constitutes a healthy meal and contribute to poor dietary choices, further exacerbating all weight loss attempts.

On the other hand, foods high in fiber, protein, and healthy fats can help keep you full and satisfied, making it easier to stick to a healthy diet. Many of us unknowingly eat products that claim to be low, fat, no sugar, or all-natural, but they do not realize that they are slowing down the fat-burning process. Ingredients matter. When you look at a product label, the nutrition panel is important, but the ingredient listing tells you the real story. Knowing the total calories of a meal does not tell you anything about what is inside the food. If you see it has chemicals, sugars, food starch, caking agents, dextrose, or maltodextrin (there are hundreds) that product will spike your insulin which means you have slowed down the possibility of weight loss for that entire day. When you see words on the label that you cannot pronounce, put the product back on the shelf.

Glucose /Blood Sugar Balance

Glucose is your body's favorite source of energy. When we eat a meal that has too much sugar or contains high glycemic foods, the insulin (hormone) levels are elevated and suddenly we are on the blood sugar rollercoaster. This is where the potential for weight gain begins. When blood sugar levels remain consistently high, all the body systems feel negatively impacted. Especially metabolism.

One of the primary ways sugars contribute to weight gain is through its effect on insulin levels. When you eat sugar, it causes blood glucose levels to rise, prompting the pancreas to release insulin. Insulin helps cells absorb glucose for energy but also plays a role in fat storage. Higher insulin levels can inhibit the body's ability to burn fat, leading to increased fat accumulation, particularly in the abdominal area. This is especially relevant for women, as hormonal fluctuations can further complicate metabolism and fat storage patterns.

Blood Sugar Rollercoaster

If you are hungry every 2 to 2 ½ hours, have trouble focusing, experience mood swings throughout the day, struggle to fall asleep (or stay asleep) at night, or battle with cravings and low energy levels, you're probably strapped into the blood sugar roller coaster.

When you eat food that spikes blood sugar fast, it tends to lead to a crash in blood sugar levels three hours later. When that happens, you get cravings, and hunger strikes again causing you to want to eat again. There is a connection between the leptin resistance mentioned earlier but the blood sugar spike is the root cause of the leptin resistance.

TIP: Our bodies are only meant to manage a teaspoon (about four grams) of sugar in the bloodstream at one time. Yes, just one teaspoon! So, you can see how the sizable portions and constant eating of sugar that are in the typical diets wreak havoc on the body.

One of the primary ways sugars contribute to weight gain is through its effect on insulin levels. When you eat sugar, it causes blood glucose levels to rise, prompting the pancreas to release insulin. Insulin helps cells absorb glucose for energy but also plays a role in fat storage. Higher insulin levels can inhibit the body's ability to burn fat, leading to increased fat accumulation, particularly in the abdominal area. This is especially relevant for women, as hormonal fluctuations can further complicate metabolism and fat storage patterns.

CHAPTER 2:
Determine Your Root Causes

When embarking on a weight loss journey, it is important to consider the factors affecting your progress. Understanding these factors or "root causes" can help you make informed decisions and achieve your weight loss goals. In this subchapter, we will explore the key factors that can influence weight loss to help you identify the principal areas that are making weight loss difficult. Root causes are imbalances in the body, or body systems, which are causing dysfunction. The dysfunction(s) are contributing to the body being reluctant to release weight. After you determine the root causes and the affected body systems, the next step is for you to address each root cause and apply the appropriate healing strategy to restore balance internally. When the body is in balance and has what it needs to thrive- weight loss becomes an amazing side effect.

As we age, the metabolism naturally slows down, making it more difficult to lose weight. It is quite common when trying to lose weight to experience the frustrating cycle of gaining and losing the same five pounds for an extended period even when staying consistent with exercise and eating patterns. Metabolism is a process by which the body's cells undergo chemical changes to convert the food we eat and drink into energy. It should also rid the body of toxic substances and provide the material cells needed for us to stay slim and healthy. But when the blood sugar is constantly high, normal metabolic processes cannot function and the consequence is effortless weight gain.

Insulin Resistance - Root Cause of Weight Gain

Insulin resistance occurs when cells in the body do not respond well to insulin, a hormone that helps regulate blood sugar levels. When we are on the blood sugar rollercoaster (up and down spiking of insulin) the cells cannot easily absorb from the blood, which causes the blood sugar levels to rise in response, the pancreas produces more insulin to try to help glucose enter the cells. Over time, the pancreas cannot keep up and the blood sugar levels continue to increase.

It is quite common for people to have insulin resistance but not realize it. Insulin resistance leads you into the direct path to pre-diabetes. If you have belly fat or feel as though any weight that you gain heads right to the belly-you can safely assume that you have insulin resistance.

Tip: You do not have to a diagnosed with pre-diabetes or Type 2 diabetes to be insulin resistant.

Insulin resistance affects people of all weights, and its symptoms can be subtle and go unnoticed. One example of this would be a person who looks healthy and slim but has a belly. Commonly referred to as "skinny fat." Signs and symptoms of insulin resistance include frequent urination, tingling in the hands and feet, fatigue, hair loss, chronic acne, sugar cravings, sugar addictions, and belly fat. The root cause of insulin resistance is elevated blood sugar. This means that the foods that you are currently eating and the nutrition plan that you typically follow are elevating blood sugar for too long and too often each day. Your body has reached its tipping point and cannot produce enough insulin to cope with the amount of glucose. So, instead of glucose going into the liver or muscle cells, the body begins to store the excess sugar as fat typically goes to the belly, hips, and thighs.

TIP: Conventional doctors recommend having an A1c glucose level of $5.7-6.2$. This is too high and not optimal for most people. Having an A1c of 5.7 or higher ensures that you will either stay on medication or always be on the borderline of prediabetes. **My recommendation is to work towards getting it below 5.2.**

Visceral Fat / Belly Fat- Root Cause

Visceral fat, often referred to as "hidden fat," is a type of body fat stored within the abdominal cavity, surrounding vital organs such as the liver, pancreas, and intestines. Unlike subcutaneous fat, which is located just beneath the skin. Visceral fat is not visible from the outside but poses significant health risks. This type of fat plays a crucial role in metabolic processes in the body and can cause health conditions including insulin resistance, type 2 diabetes, heart disease, and certain cancers. Understanding visceral fat is essential to adopting an effective nutrition plan aimed at reducing this specific type of fat.

The measurement of visceral fat is particularly important as it provides insight into one's overall health. While body mass index (BMI) is a commonly used metric to assess body weight relative to height, it does not distinguish between types of fat. For women, a higher proportion of visceral fat can lead to hormonal imbalances that may affect reproductive health, contribute to weight gain, and increase the risk of chronic diseases. For men, a common scenario is the development of diabetes or heart disease. Therefore, focusing on visceral fat loss can be a more effective approach to achieving long-term health and wellness goals.

Many factors contribute to the accumulation of visceral fat. Genetics plays a significant role, but lifestyle choices such as diet, physical activity, and stress management are equally important. Diets high in refined carbohydrates, sugars, and unhealthy fats can promote the storage of visceral fat. Additionally, sedentary lifestyles and chronic stress can increase cortisol levels, which can lead to fat accumulation around the abdomen. Recognizing these factors is crucial for developing targeted nutrition plans that address the root causes of visceral fat gain.

Effective strategies for visceral fat loss often incorporate balanced nutrition, regular exercise, and lifestyle modifications. A diet rich in whole foods, including fruits, vegetables, lean proteins, and healthy fats, can help combat visceral fat accumulation. Incorporating physical activity, particularly strength training and high-intensity interval training (HIIT), can also enhance fat-burning and improve metabolic health.

TIP # 1 To increase the potential for visceral fat loss each week, take 2 Tablespoons of Braggs Apple Cider vinegar every day.

TIP # 2   When you have a meal that has carbs or a "cheat meal" take 1- tablespoon of ACV before the meal. It will minimize the blood sugar impact (glucose spikes) by 30 %.

The trouble with belly fat is that it is not limited to the layer of padding just below the skin called subcutaneous fat. Belly fat also includes visceral fat. And that lies deep inside the abdomen and surrounds the internal organs.

Regardless of a person's overall weight, having a large amount of belly fat raises the risk of:

- High blood pressure.
- An unhealthy amount of fat in the blood.
- Sleep apnea.

Heart disease.

- High blood sugar and diabetes. Certain cancers.
- Stroke.
- Fatty liver.
- Early death from any cause.

Measuring your middle

To see if your belly fat is a concern, measure your waist:

- Stand and place a tape measure around your bare stomach, just above your hip bone.
- Pull the tape measure until it fits snugly but does not push into the skin. Make sure the tape measure is level all the way around.
- Relax, exhale, and measure your waist. Do not suck in your stomach as you measure.

For women, a waist measurement of more than thirty-five inches (89 centimeters) signals an unhealthy amount of belly fat and is a marker for insulin resistance which leads to diabetes or other serious health problems. For men, the waist measurement of forty inches or more. In general, though, the greater the waist measurement, the higher the health risks. Unfortunately, when it comes to fat loss, we cannot tell our bodies where we do (and do not) want the fat to go, but the goal is to strive to eat well and choose the best foods we can.

Unhealthy Gut- Root Cause

A healthy gut is crucial for weight loss and lifelong weight management. If you are experiencing a lot of daily symptoms while trying to lose weight such as bloating, gas, heartburn, sugar cravings, joint pain brain fog, fatigue, or headaches, this could be a sign that you have digestive dysfunction which is affecting your body's ability to digest and absorb

nutrients. When we eat food, the food is processed in the gut, broken down into molecules, and absorbed into our blood or sent out to the garbage disposal. Bowel distress can develop- such as leaky gut, irritable bowel syndrome, and slowed intestinal transit. Diet is the direct link.

Is Your Food Medicine or Poison to Your Gut

Bad gut bugs grow for two reasons: not eating enough of the food that feeds the good guys and eating too many gut-busting foods. The biggest culprit is gluten. Modern wheat has powerful inflammatory proteins called gliadin that create a leaky gut. Glyphosate, the weed killer, is sprayed on wheat at harvest to dry out. Your morning Cheerios has more glyphosate than vitamin B12 and vitamin D added to the cereal. Why is that bad? Aside from being a known carcinogen, glyphosate destroys your microbiome. Other common gut-busting foods include sugar and starch. The bad guys love it just like you do. It promotes the overgrowth of toxic bacteria and yeast, and it is the reason for getting a "food baby" after a meal. Refined oils, which make up about 10 percent of our calories, also lead to leaky gut and trigger something called metabolic endotoxemia. In other words, our metabolism is constantly poisoned because of toxic byproducts of bad bacteria, leading to obesity and type 2 diabetes. Omega 3 fats do the opposite.

TIP: If you feel your root cause of resistant weight loss is gut health, your first step should be to detox your body from sugar and see a healthcare professional to work on a gut healing protocol or reach out to me via email to schedule a consultation. After you begin to heal your gut, your body will have an easier time releasing the excess weight.

Leaky Gut Syndrome

Leaky gut is one of the most common root causes of weight loss that I see in my patients, but conventional medicine doctors do not address or acknowledge it. Glucose spikes can significantly increase the potential to develop leaky gut syndrome inflammation, which is one of the processes set off by insulin glucose spikes, can cause holes in the gut lining which then allow toxins (sugars, alcohol, processed foods) to go through the gut wall into the bloodstream. This leads to food allergies, autoimmune, hormone imbalance, joint pain, and weight gain. Mental health issues are also linked to a leaky gut. Anxiety is the most common. Anxiety is a common eating behavior that contributes to overeating and weight gain. A healthy gut means weight loss becomes much less of a struggle.

Toxicity In the Body- Root Cause

When you hear the word, "detox," you may think of drug or alcohol rehab or fad "cleansing" diets. But our body "detoxes" all the time, and it keeps us alive and healthy. Imagine if your toilet backs up for a week or if your sink is clogged up for a few days. It is not too pretty. The same things happen in your body if your detoxification system fails. If your liver fails, you cannot process waste and you end up yellow (jaundice) and needing a liver transplant. If your kidneys stop working, you cannot process water waste, get extremely sick, and will die in a week or two without dialysis. If your colon is clogged up it leads to serious problems. Thankfully, our biology is designed to process waste and toxins through our intricate detoxification system. The process of detoxification can be hindered by an overload of toxic insults, such as processed food, too much sugar and starch, and environmental toxins, among many others. Your detoxification systems also require a host of nutrients to function optimally.

The scary reality is that most physicians are not trained adequately in this part of our physiology. Many doctors will tell you that the body knows how to get rid of chemicals and other toxins, which is true, however, your detoxification system cannot keep up with the onslaught of modern-day chemicals, toxins, and other insults we face at every turn. So, unfortunately, both the diagnosis and treatment of impaired detoxification are rarely made. Many of our common diseases are linked to an overload of toxins including heart disease, diabetes, cancer, obesity, and dementia. Environmental toxins, also referred to as obesogens, cause weight gain. Sadly, many of us are toxic waste dumps but do not realize it. More than eighty thousand chemicals have been introduced into the environment since the Industrial Revolution, and most have never been evaluated for safety. They cause inflammation, and oxidative stress, damage the mitochondria, disrupt our gut function, create hormonal imbalances, and overload our detoxification systems. This leads to the body becoming resistant to releasing weight.

Tip: Do a total body detox to rid the body of its toxic burden- one to two times a year.

Hormone Imbalance- Root Cause

Hormonal changes can affect metabolism and appetite, making it easier to gain weight and harder to lose it. It is important to work with a healthcare provider to monitor hormone levels and address any imbalances that may be hindering weight loss progress. If your hormone blood comes back in "normal ranges. "But keep in mind that lab ranges are very general. If you are rating low or at the high end of a range, that means your body is not functioning as optimally as it could be and there are potential imbalances that need to be investigated. When you feel something is off, it probably is. Trust your gut feelings and dig deeper for more information. Your doctor should feel like a partner or advocate on your weight loss and health journey.

For example, menopause can lead to a decrease in estrogen levels, which can affect metabolism and lead to weight gain. By understanding how hormones affect weight loss, you can adjust your nutrition, exercise, and natural medicine to support those natural processes instead of starting with prescription medication.

Stress and sleep are important factors to consider when trying to lose weight. Chronic stress can lead to overeating and weight gain, while lack of sleep can disrupt hormone levels and metabolism, making it harder to lose weight. It is important to incorporate stress management techniques and ensure you are getting enough quality sleep to support your weight loss efforts.

Both men and women can develop a sluggish metabolism. This affects how we lose and maintain weight as we age. One of the root causes of sluggish metabolism is our history of dieting attempts. Our food habits during our high school years and throughout our thirties play a role in damaging metabolic function. Example: Many women have tried many different diets throughout their lives which either involve some type of processed food that is store-bought, or a weight loss program that offers packaged "weight loss food."

Adrenal Fatigue and Inflammation- Root Cause

Adrenal fatigue is one of the most common conditions that I see in my office each week. Especially in women. Adrenal health is intricately linked to insulin resistance, a condition that often emerges with age and is exacerbated by chronic inflammation. When adrenal function has been compromised, the body's ability to regulate blood sugar levels can become impaired, leading to increased insulin resistance. As previously mentioned, insulin resistance- in and of itself- is a root cause of weight gain. Add adrenal fatigue and chronic inflammation to the mix and you. have a recipe for major roadblocks to any weight loss plan.

One of the significant consequences of chronic inflammation is its impact on the adrenal glands, which are responsible for producing hormones that help the adrenal glands become overworked due to the body's constant inflammatory state, leading to a condition called adrenal fatigue. This condition is characterized by a decline in adrenal function, resulting in symptoms such as fatigue, mood swings, and difficulty managing weight. As the adrenal glands struggle to cope with ongoing inflammation, their ability to produce essential hormones like cortisol may become compromised, further exacerbating health issues.

Symptoms of Adrenal Fatigue

Adrenal fatigue, a term often used to describe a collection of symptoms related to the overwhelmed adrenal glands, is increasingly recognized because of chronic inflammation and stress. Understanding the symptoms of adrenal fatigue is crucial, particularly as it can significantly impact overall health and weight management. The adrenal glands play a vital role in the body's response to stress, and when they become exhausted, a myriad of physical and psychological symptoms can manifest.

One of the primary indicators of adrenal fatigue is persistent fatigue that does not improve with rest. Clients typically report feeling drained despite a full night's sleep, which can lead to a reliance on caffeine or stimulants to get through the day. This chronic tiredness is intense fatigue and is accompanied by a reduced ability to manage stress, leading to feelings of overwhelm in situations that previously felt manageable. It is also important to consider the fatigue. The fatigue is different than just being sluggish in the afternoon because you need a sugar boost. Adrenal fatigue typically does not respond well to sugar, meaning that it does not help with energy levels. The link between adrenal fatigue and chronic inflammation amplifies these symptoms, as inflammation can. exacerbate feelings of exhaustion and contribute to a cycle of fatigue and stress. In addition to fatigue, individuals may experience mood swings, irritability, or anxiety. The adrenal glands are responsible for the production of hormones such as cortisol, which regulate stress responses. When the adrenal glands are fatigued, cortisol levels may become imbalanced, leading to emotional instability. This hormonal disruption can also affect sleep quality, resulting in insomnia or restless nights, further compounding the fatigue and emotional distress. Consider this: Emotional eating is common with people who have adrenal fatigue in that is looking for quick energy and it drives the cravings for sugars. Tip: If you heal the adrenal fatigue, the emotional eating events will begin to lessen.

Chronic inflammation has also been linked to insulin resistance, a condition where the body's cells become less responsive to insulin, leading to elevated blood sugar levels. This relationship is particularly concerning for individuals over forty, as the risk of developing insulin resistance and type 2 diabetes increases with age. Elevated levels of inflammatory markers, such as C-reactive protein (CRP) and interleukin-6- 6 (IL-6), have played a role in the development of insulin resistance. As the body struggles to maintain normal blood sugar levels, it can lead to weight gain, particularly around the abdominal area, which is associated with a higher risk of cardiovascular disease and other health complications.

Weight management can become increasingly challenging when chronic inflammation is present, as it can create a vicious cycle that perpetuates both weight gain and inflammation. The body's response to chronic inflammation often includes an increase in fat storage, particularly visceral fat, and is linked to hormonal imbalances. This can lead to further inflammation, creating a feedback loop that makes it difficult for individuals to lose weight or maintain a healthy weight. For those over 40, addressing chronic inflammation is essential not only for weight management but also for preventing other age-related health issues.

Holistic To Healing Adrenal Fatigue.

The most important thing to do to heal adrenal fatigue is to adjust your nutrition. It is crucial to get the sugars out and to have a steady flow of nutrient-dense food throughout the day. High Protein, healthy fats, and quality protein-fat snacks. You want to think of food as your medicine to nourish and support the adrenal glands and it will not take long for you to notice a difference in energy levels. I also recommend supplementing adaptogenic herbs such as ashwagandha and Rhodiola rosea to my patients to support the adrenal glands. These natural remedies have been used for centuries in traditional medicine to enhance stress resilience and support adrenal function. Adaptogens help the body adapt to stressors, which can be particularly beneficial for individuals facing the dual challenges of chronic inflammation and adrenal fatigue. Incorporating these herbs into a daily routine may foster a more balanced physiological response to stress, leading to improved energy levels and weight stability.

While supplements and natural remedies can provide significant benefits, they work best when paired with a nutritious diet. Start with your nutrition adjustments first/ See how your body responds then incorporate them in a supplement. Addressing chronic inflammation and supporting adrenal health requires a comprehensive strategy that considers all aspects of well-being. As you navigate these complex interconnections, the right combination of supplements and lifestyle adjustments can lead to improved health outcomes and get the scale moving in the right direction again.

Fake Food

When we ingest artificial(fake) foods, it "confuses" the metabolism and disrupts the natural flow of the metabolic processes. Over time, the metabolism will not function at peak performance and fat burning becomes difficult. It is common for people who have done well on Keto to suddenly stop losing weight/ This happens because their body has reached the point that they must address the metabolic issues, unhealthy gut, and emotional ties to food. Our metabolism functions and burns fat efficiently when we give it the right fuel to burn.

How Do Prescription Medications Impact Weight Loss

I am certain that none of us would want to live in a world without access to lifesaving medications or medications that are necessary. But it should not be your only available choice. If you feel a "nudge" in your gut that you do not want to take medications, investigate your options. An example of this would be women who struggle with weight issues and have high cholesterol and/or blood pressure issues. This is a tough cycle to be in. Nutrition and diet can usually help with improving blood work, but the medications may also be contributing to resistant weight loss because the body takes in medications as "foreign" and thereby disrupts the metabolic process and makes weight loss more difficult.

FACT: There are effective natural medicines that can work as well as statins and various forms of blood pressure medications but unfortunately, doctors only give the option for prescriptions.

Weight Loss Medications- Is This the Best Option for You

Semaglutide helps to lower blood sugar levels and regulates insulin, which is crucial for people with type 2 diabetes. This drug also imitates a hormone called glucagon-like peptide-1 that is naturally produced in our intestines, and it limits appetite by signaling to our bodies that we do feel full. It has been effective with weight loss and people with obesity. Medicine helps to make the person feel fuller and faster.

Clients who started seeing me after taking Semaglutide reported side effects including blood clots behind the eyes, intense joint pain, dizziness, and joint pain. When they come off the drug, they still have the old habits to deal with that made them want to start the drug in the first place. Additionally, emotional eating behaviors become a huge catalyst in gaining weight back because they have not dealt with the issues that made them gain weight in the first place.

If you are considering or are currently taking weight loss medications, ask yourself, "Is it sustainable?" What will your life look like 10 years from now? Will you be able to maintain the weight loss and afford the injections?" A key consideration is what will be the long-term effects of the medications. If you are confused as to how to manage nutrition, lifestyle, food sensitivity, or emotional eating behaviors, it will feel worse after you stop taking the medication.

Many natural supplements work like Ozempic. Ozempic is a GLP-1 receptor agonist. This class of drugs helps to increase a gut hormone called "incretin." Incretin has an action on the pancreas in secreting insulin helping to stabilize blood sugar levels, trick your brain, and decrease your appetite. Yes, it does work to release weight, but we do not know the long-term consequences of taking the injections.

Natural Alternatives to Ozempic-No Side Effects

Quercetin can increase the GLP1- just like the drugs do, but it is natural with no side effects.

EGCG Is an antioxidant and contains caffeine and green tea. It targets belly fat.

Panax Ginseng is an adaptogenic herbal medicine that stabilizes insulin levels and regulates blood glucose levels and cortisol levels (stress hormone).

Cinnamon - Cinnamon stabilizes blood sugar.

Curcumin is a natural anti-inflammatory and stabilizes blood sugar.

Maca is an adaptogenic herb and it helps to manage stress and our reactions to stress. It also gives us energy and stamina and is particularly effective if you take it before a workout.

Calcium- In a low calcium state our bodies go into a state called lipogenesis (the making of more fat) which comprises any weight loss efforts if you are not getting enough absorbable calcium.

Natural Metabolic Enhancers

L-Carnitine: An amino acid that helps in fat metabolism.

Alpha-Lipoic Acid: An antioxidant that supports energy metabolism and helps in managing blood sugar levels

Bloodwork To Request from Your Doctor

Is your doctor checking all the appropriate lab work at your annual visit? Many doctors order the bare minimum and do not check enough things to develop the full picture to determine if you are truly healthy.

TIP: Remember, if your goal is weight loss, you are on the hunt for all the imbalances in your body to get to the root cause of insulin resistance and metabolic dysfunction. You need all the information- and you have a right to ask for it.

BMP, CBC - Lipid panel – tests bare minimum looks at kidney function, fasting level, electrolytes, blood cell count, HDL cholesterol, triglycerides, and gross infection or inflammation.

A1c – you can have a normal fasting blood sugar on your labs but still be pre-diabetic- A1c immediately detects prediabetes.

CMP- Comprehensive Metabolic Panel, also checks Liver function.

CBC w/Diff- Complete Blood Panel

C- Peptide – an excellent proxy marker for how much insulin your pancreas must make to deal with the amount of carbs you are eating. Elevated levels signify early diabetes (even if fasting glucose and A1c are in the normal range)

D-25 – Doctors order Vit D 1 but Vit D 25 is best to detect deficiency.

DHEA-S -Looks at the overall adrenal gland.

ESR (sed rate) – a marker for chronic inappropriate inflammation

Ferritin – relates inflammation and hyperinsulinemia.

Fasting Insulin – checks if the pancreas is secreting too much insulin-

a marker for metabolic syndrome.

GGT – checks damage to liver

Homocysteine- an excellent indicator of b12 and overall inflammation in the body

CRP Reactive Protein -if elevated there is inflammation somewhere in your body.

Lipid Panel – triglycerides

Magnesium – tests for deficiency

Phosphorus – tests for deficiency

TSH-Thyroid Stimulating Hormone - a snapshot of thyroid function to make sure it is functioning ok.

Urinalysis – looks for ketones and signs of infection or damage in the body.

Consider asking for these tests at least once a year. Your doctor should be your partner and health advocate, providing you with information so that you can make the best decisions you can for your health. Conventional doctors are only given the option to take 1 semester of nutrition in medical school. The takeaway is to understand that most health conditions respond to personalized nutrition adjustments and there is absolutely no need to take prescription medication.

If your doctor is not open to natural alternatives consider expanding your health care team so that you can make the best decision for your health. Many people face the challenge of deciding whether to pursue other doctors. Be diplomatic about it and bring the list of labs that you would like to run if they cannot give you or are not willing to work in partnership with you on your journey to your best health- find another doctor. If you cannot find anyone in your area, please contact me through DrLorimahler.com and we can arrange a virtual meeting consultation.

Challenges Faced by Women Over 50

As women age, our bodies undergo various changes that can make weight loss more challenging. We often face unique obstacles when it comes to achieving our weight loss goals. These challenges can range from hormonal fluctuations to a slower metabolism, making it harder to shed excess pounds and maintain a healthy weight. One common challenge is hormonal changes, particularly during menopause. Fluctuating hormone levels can lead to weight gain, especially belly fat around midsection. Additionally, hormonal changes can also impact energy levels and mood, making it harder to stay motivated and stick to a healthy eating and exercise routine. Fluctuating hormone levels typically mean blood sugar levels are part of the problem. When we experience hot "flashes", which could be a high blood sugar response from something we have eaten.

Tip: Tracking daily food intake during the times that hot flashes are common can help identify any foods that could be contributing to the fluctuating hormones. Excessive rises in blood sugar can cause a flush or heated feeling in the body. It may not be a hot flash caused by menopause.

CHAPTER 3:
Preparing for Sustainable Weight Loss

Setting goals is a crucial aspect of any weight loss journey. It gives you a solid target to work towards. Without clear goals in mind, it can be easy to lose motivation and direction. By setting specific goals, you can create a roadmap to success in your weight loss efforts. These goals provide a sense of purpose and help you stay focused on your ultimate objectives.

One of the key benefits of setting goals is that it allows you to track your progress and celebrate your achievements along the way. Every inch or pound lost is an enormous success! Start by breaking down large goals into smaller, more manageable milestones, you can stay motivated and see tangible results. Staying motivated throughout the process can feel incredibly challenging. Especially if you do not see the scale moving the way you want, achieving small, but important goals, will give you a sense of accomplishment, boost confidence, and provide the motivation needed to continue making healthy choices.

Setting goals will also help you stay accountable to yourself and others. Create a network of encouragement and accountability by sharing your goals with friends, family, or a support group. Knowing that others are

rooting for your success can provide the extra push needed to stay on track, even when faced with challenges or setbacks.

Additionally, setting small goals may help you to prioritize your time and resources. By identifying what is profoundly important to you, and aligning your goals with your values, you can make more intentional choices about spending your time and energy. This can lead to greater efficiency and effectiveness in your weight loss efforts.

Structured Goal Setting

When setting a weight loss goal, it is important to be specific about what you want to achieve. Instead of saying, "I want to lose weight," try setting a goal such as, "I want to lose 10 pounds in the next three months." This gives you a clear target to work towards and helps you stay focused on your ultimate objective.

Measurable goals are key to tracking your progress and staying motivated. By setting specific targets, such as losing a certain number of pounds or inches, you can easily measure your success along the way. Be sure to take your measurements every 10 days or so. You want to have a variety of ways to see your progress. You will experience weight loss on the scale for some weeks, and in other weeks you will lose inches. You want a mix of both! This means that your body's composition is changing and that is an exceptionally good thing. There may be weeks when you do not see much happening on the scale, but you *feel weight loss* and you go down the size of your clothes. Learn to tune in and notice how your body is changing. Look at yourself naked in the mirror so that you can *see the* changes happening. I know that it sounds hard to do but this can help you stay on track and adjust your plan as needed to ensure you reach your goal. It requires a mindset shift from the scale to how your body *feels. Slow and steady weight loss is best to achieve sustainable weight loss.* Losing more than three pounds each week feels great at the time, but you want to be sure the weight loss is sustainable and not easily regained. Setting unattainable goals can lead to frustration and disappointment while setting achievable goals can boost your confidence and keep you motivated to continue your weight loss journey. A good average weight loss each week is 2-3 pounds If a consistent exercise program is part of your week, then your weight loss will be on the higher end.

TIP: If you are a member of the "I have dieted most of my life and still can't lose weight club," you should know by now what makes you lose your motivation. By setting goals that are relevant to your lifestyle, preferences, and values, you are more likely to stay committed and motivated to achieve them. Finally, setting time for your goals ensures that you have a sense of urgency and accountability. By giving yourself a deadline, you are more likely to stay focused and dedicated to reaching your weight loss goals. Remember, goal setting is a powerful tool that can help you stay on track and achieve success in your weight loss journey.

Tracking Progress

Tracking progress is an essential aspect of achieving your weight loss goals. By monitoring your progress, you can see how far you have come and stay motivated to keep going. One of the most effective ways to track your progress is by keeping a food journal. Write down everything you eat and drink throughout the day, along with the portion sizes. Even the things that are not on your nutrition plan. This will help you identify any patterns or habits that may be hindering your weight loss efforts. A valuable tool for tracking progress is measuring your body composition. This includes tracking your weight, body fat percentage, and measurements of key areas such as your waist, hips, and thighs. By regularly measuring these metrics, you can see changes in your body composition over time and adjust your diet and exercise routine.

Weight loss is not just about the scale number, eating clean, and exercising. It is about healthy body composition. A healthy body has lean muscle, proper hydration, and a healthy fat percentage so you can feel your absolute best. In addition to physical measurements, it is also important to track your fitness progress. Keep a log of your workouts, including the type of exercise, duration, and intensity. You can also track your strength and endurance levels by recording the amount of weight you lift or the number of repetitions you can do. By monitoring your fitness progress, you can see improvements in your strength and stamina, which is just as rewarding as seeing changes in your body composition.

One of the benefits of tracking progress is that it allows you to celebrate your achievements along the way. Whether you want to lose 10 or 100 pounds, fit into a smaller size, or run a faster mile, each milestone is a reason to celebrate. Acknowledge your hard work and dedication and reward yourself for reaching your goals. This positive reinforcement will help you stay motivated and committed to your weight loss journey.

Tracking progress is a crucial component of successful weight loss. You are building good habits along the way. Keep a food journal, measure your body composition, track your fitness progress, and celebrate your achievements, so you can stay on track and reach your goals each week.

STOP WEIGHING YOURSELF EVERYDAY

There are several things you can do to combat a slower metabolism which should include nutrition adjustments, and an enjoyable, consistent exercise routine. Consider using a food scale to monitor your portion sizes as well as a body composition scale to check your weight once a week. Avoid weighing yourself every day. This will only set you up for the mind games that many of us have put ourselves through when we step on the scale and do not see weight loss. Remember, the scale number is just an indicator of the fluid balance in the body at the time you weigh. Fluid balance changes every day. The best way to gauge your weight loss is to weigh the same time each week, in the same clothes every 7 days. This will be your true weight loss result.

Getting a good body fat composition scale is a valuable tool to use on your weight loss journey. It will help you to determine your fat loss each week. It is important to know what you are losing. Are you losing fat, muscle, or water weight? When the scale number does go down you want to know for sure that you are not losing muscle, because muscle mass helps to burn fat. The goal is to think about your long-term goal. Focus on losing body fat and on maintaining or building lean muscle mass over time. Despite these challenges, you may also feel you have tried everything under the sun to lose weight, but nothing works long-term Every person who is struggling with weight issues has a diverse set of root cause(s)" as to why the weight loss is not happening. Think of your root causes as the keys to reaching your weight loss goal.

TIP: When I was going through my weight loss journey, I was addicted to weighing myself every single morning. My solution was to make my husband hide the scale until it was time for my actual weight-in.

Understanding the unique obstacles that you continually find yourself dealing with is part of your roadmap to your perfect weight. You are battling the same issues (habits and eating behaviors) for a reason. With the right mindset, support system, strategies in place, and a better understanding of your body - you can achieve a slim and strong body that reflects your inner strength and resilience

Stop Eating as Soon as You Feel Comfortably Full

Quite often, when I am working with a patient, they will express concern that they don't know what it feels like to feel "comfortably full." This is quite common, especially for people who have weight to lose.

From a hunger perspective, our body is supposed to signal us when it feels full. (leptin signaling). When the hunger hormones (leptin and ghrelin) are out of not doing their job, we do not get the memo that we have had enough, and we can eat far beyond what we require. Especially if we are eating low-nutrient-dense food.

Comfortably full means that you could take another bite, but you do not because you feel you have had enough. This is how we are meant to eat. The hormones will reset as you eat the right portions throughout the day and retrain your digestive tract to understand what a true portion should be.

TIP: Follow the tips for resetting leptin signaling and use the appropriate serving sizes for 2 weeks. You will start to notice that your body will start to feel fuller much quicker than you used to.

How To Stop the Uncontrollable Hunger

The science of hunger and satiety are physiological processes. They are controlled by your hormones and your brain stem and are hardwired into your physiology to tell you that you are either hungry or full. There are ways that you can hack these hormones and put them in a sweet spot so that you can appropriately not feel hungry for hours or feel appropriately full after eating a meal. I refer to this feeling as comfortably full. The following tips will help you to stop yo-yo dieting and help you to make concrete changes for successful maintenance.

Leptin, ghrelin, cortisol, neuropeptide Y, Peptide YY, Cholecystokinin, and GLP-1

How to Stop Overeating and Reset Leptin Levels

Stop eating all the sugar and sweeteners. Natural, artificial sweeteners, natural sugars, fruit agave, sodas, and sweetened coffees. You are still raising your insulin levels even though you are not eating actual sugar.

Stop eating all the grains. Grains are a little better than eating sugar but not much. They have the same effect on the body as eating actual sugar.

Stop eating as soon as you feel comfortably full.

Stop eating baked goods. Baked goods reignite old eating behaviors and reawaken sugar addictions.

Control your stress. Learn strategies to control your stress and manage cortisol levels

Get good sleep. Your body needs to be repaired and recover. if it does not you are more susceptible to cravings daily.

Stop snacking in between meals. Wait at least 3 hours between meals or snacks to avoid excessive glucose spikes.

Eat enough healthy fats. Eating fat does not make you fat. The macronutrient fat helps turn on the hunger hormone to your sweet spot so you can go longer without snacking.

Eat more protein, Protein will never make you fat. It turns off hunger and helps you stop sugar cravings.

Eat Fruit with a protein and a healthy fat. This will ensure that the fruit sugar does not cause a significant glucose spike.

Tip: It is also important to lower your stress levels and turn off your blue screens at least one hour before bed. Find relaxing meditative music or gentle hypnosis to completely quiet your mind before you try to sleep.

CHAPTER 4:
Nutrition- Food Is Medicine

Nutrition is the key to successful, lifelong weight management. To achieve and maintain a healthy weight, it is important to follow a personalized approach to your diet. A balanced diet is different for everyone and should consist of a variety of foods including fruits, vegetables, lean proteins, and healthy fats. By incorporating a wide range of nutrients into your daily meals, you can ensure that your body is getting all the essential vitamins and minerals it needs to function optimally.

One of the key components of a balanced diet is portion control. It is important to eat the right amount of food to meet your body's energy needs. By being mindful of portion sizes and listening to your body's hunger cues, you can prevent overeating and avoid unnecessary weight gain. Additionally, eating smaller, more frequent meals throughout the day will keep your metabolism revved up and prevent you from feeling overly hungry, which can lead to unhealthy food choices.

How Does Whole Food Nutrition Help Us Reach Our Weight Loss Goal

In addition to eating a variety of foods, it is important to pay attention to the quality of the food you are consuming. Choose the best quality food you can. Choose whole, minimally processed foods whenever possible because they are typically higher in nutrients and lower in added sugars, unhealthy fats, and preservatives.

Food As Medicine to Our Body

In naturopathic medicine, we recognize that the body is not organized into different specialties. We look at the body as an integrated unit.

What drives all excess weight and disease imbalances is the fundamental networks underlying all diseases. Networks that are all dynamically interacting every moment with your lifestyle, disease triggers, food intake, and genes. Most diseases stem from imbalances and toxins in seven interconnected systems. Heal the body's affected body systems, and in most cases, you do not have to treat the actual disease, and weight loss becomes a side effect. If you give your body what it needs, it can heal itself.

Fake Food

The definition of fake food is anything that food manufacturers have artificially tampered with by manufacturers- anything that comes in a bag, box, or can. When we ingest fake) foods, it "confuses" metabolism and disrupts the natural flow of the metabolic processes. Over time, the metabolism will not function at peak performance and fat burning becomes difficult. One example of this would be the Keto diet. Yes, it is highly effective for weight loss, but many people are also adding keto products which is just more processed food. In my experience, people stop losing on Keto because at some point they must address the metabolic issues, unhealthy gut, and emotional ties to food.

Body Systems and What They Do

1. Assimilation (digestion, absorption, microbiome, digestive

2. Defense & Repair (immune, inflammation, infections, microbiota)

3. Energy (energy regulation, mitochondrial function)

4. Biotransformation & Elimination (toxicity, detoxification)

5. Transport (cardiovascular, lymphatic system)

6. Communication (endocrine, neurotransmitters, immune messengers)

7. Structural integrity (from subcellular membranes to musculoskeletal structure)

Food is the biggest lever to impact on all these systems. The wrong food harms each system and the right food helps optimize each system. The right food regulates the health of your microbiome, your immune system and reduces levels of inflammation, and oxidative stress, and improves your energy systems. Food balances your hormones and brain chemistry, supports detoxification, and improves the function and health of our circulatory and lymphatic systems, it even provides the raw materials for every cell, muscle, tissue, organ, and bone in your body.

While most doctors have not seen the power of food, mostly because they are not trained in medical school on how to use food as medicine, I have seen miracles over decades and so have many other naturopathic doctors. Except they are not miracles. They are the result of applying the latest. Advances in understanding how our bodies work with holistic nutrition and natural medicine. Autoimmune diseases disappear, depression vanishes, migraines evaporate, psoriasis and eczema clear up, Alzheimer's patients improve their memory, and type 2 diabetes can be reversed in as little as 30 days. These are abnormalities or spontaneous remissions, but reproducible results based on applying food as medicine with the model of naturopathic medicine. When we apply the healing power of nature's nutrients, (whole, nutrient-dense food, healing begins.

There is no other activity you do every day that has more power to change your biology than what you eat. You ingest pounds of foreign material into your body every day. If all calories were the same, it would not matter what you eat, but this is not the case. Food carries information molecules, instructions, and code that programs your biology with every bite for better or worse. It fuels you with nourishment and stimulates the body to release excess weight.

Industrial food drives inflammation, oxidative stress, imbalances in hormone and brain chemistry, damages your microbiome, and changes your gene expression to turn on disease-causing genes. Whole-nutrient and phytonutrient-rich food does the opposite, While we all need certain macronutrients to achieve our best health, I have found that this is the wrong approach for weight loss. When new clients begin working with me, they quickly realize that my approach is different than anything they have heard before. I factor in the timing of meals, portion control based on the needs of their body, and food combing principles to create fat-burning meals and stabilize blood sugar.

Start with a baseline portion of food and then continue to adjust based on your hunger at each meal. This approach helps to reset that portion size "switch" (ghrelin and leptin) that we all have but often ignore. Portion control means that you feel fully satisfied and stop eating on your own. The goal is to customize your macronutrient baseline to not only nourish your body but also facilitate health and weight loss. I gauge my patient's progress by how quickly they get hungry. In other words, you should be able to eat every 3 to 4 hours and feel ready to eat a snack or a meal. If it is a properly combined meal or snack based on my guidelines which I will share shortly. You may be thinking that it sounds strange to eat so often when weight loss is the goal, but this is an area that requires a shift in thinking. It is a good sign when your body gets hungry (if you are eating the right thing). It is an indication that your body is doing an excellent job at digesting, assimilating, and absorbing the food you are eating. If you do not get hungry for 6 to 7 hours, this typically means the food is sitting in your colon and not being utilized as fuel. This and creates toxicity in the body sets you on the path to disease.

Why Is Protein Important

Build- Protein is an important building block of bones, muscles, cartilage, and skin. Your hair, skin, and nails are composed of protein.

Repair. Your body uses it to repair tissue. Red blood cells contain a protein compound that carries oxygen throughout the body. This helps supply your body with the nutrients it needs.

Digest. About half of the dietary protein, you need each day goes into making enzymes, which aid in digesting food and making new cells and body chemicals. (This is why a set macronutrient goal does not work for everyone).

Regulate. Protein plays a huge role in hormone balance.

Protein also

1) Speeds up recovery after exercise and or injury.

2). Reduces muscle loss.

3). Building lean muscle mass.

4). Helps us maintain a healthy weight.

5). Satiates hunger and stops sugar cravings.

Recommendation Base Protein Servings to Start With:

Use a food scale to measure.

Intake for Women -Start with 4 to 5 Serving

Intake for Men- Start with 5- 7 ounces.

Healthy Fats

There are a lot of myths surrounding the recommendation of eating high-fat foods, and whether are not we should eat them. (You might remember the low-fat dieting crazes of yesteryear). You must eat the right amount of healthy fats. All fats are not created equal.

Why is Fat Important?

Fat is an energy source: When you limit carb intake and increase your fat intake your body recovers its ability to burn fat for energy reducing fat deposits and reducing your weight.

Fat helps you feel full. Feeling full means snacking less.

Fat helps regulate blood sugar. Fat slows down the release of glucose into the blood, which helps to keep your blood sugar from spiking or crashing- with an additional bonus of reducing sugar cravings.

Fat carries flavor. More flavorful food is more satisfying, which can help curb snacking and overeating.

Recommendations for Healthy Fat and Carbs- Serving Size

Serving size for women - I tablespoon

Serving size for men - 2 tablespoons

Vegetable Carbohydrates – Non-starchy vegetables are high in fiber and have all the essential vitamins and minerals that you need.

Serving size for women – 2 cups plus unlimited greens

Serving Size for men – 3 cups plus unlimited greens

Tip: As you work toward your weight loss goal, starchy vegetables can be added back in slowly / small portions. Start with ½ cup cooked Begin planning your meals based on the above serving sizes. The key is to stop eating when you feel comfortably full. This amount is different for each of us. It will take some time for you to connect with the feeling of being 'comfortably full." Be sure to reset your leptin signaling- this will help you to start naturally feeling full. Eating this way is not about eating. keto although you are minimizing the carbs until your blood sugar stabilizes. If you go through life thinking carbs are the devil, then you will always feel restricted and that is not sustainable.

How To Eat

1) Eat through the day 3 to 5 times.

2) The first meal of the day should be a high-protein meal.

3) Be sure to add your healthy fat. Healthy fat will not make you fat unless you are eating a huge volume at meal or snack time.

4) Avoid "drinking" your calories. Quality protein shakes are ok. Avoid soda, flavored water coffees, Starbucks, and Duncan Donuts.

5) Wait at least three hours between meals or snacks. Your body needs three full hours to digest the contents in the stomach. If you eat three hours before, the digestion process stops, and you slow down the weight loss for that day.

6). Best Fruits to have- Start with apples, berries and grapefruits. During your first and second weeks, have up to four servings of fruit in the week. Add it you your protein meal.

Start with one serving up to four times in the first several weeks. Best Food for Weight Loss and Resetting the Body

Lean Proteins – All white fish, salmon, shrimp, 95% lean red meat, Greek yogurt, part skim cheese (no added starch or caking agents), turkey, chicken, and lamb.

Healthy fats -Avocado, olive oil, coconut oil, avocado oil, 100% grass-fed butter, farm-raised eggs, tuna (fresh), all seeds, all nuts.

Favorite dressing recommendation – Primal Kitchen, G.H Hughes

Vegetables (Carbohydrates)

Unlimited Greens – All greens and herbs

Fruit Serving - Apples, berries, and grapefruit. 1 medium or 1 cup of grapefruit with a meal or snack

TIP: Peanuts and almonds tend to slow down weight loss in some people. If you are not losing weight or stopped losing weight – be sure to eat nuts with a serving of protein. Nuts by themselves tend to slow down weight loss for some people. In my experience, I have seen clients lose 30 or 40 pounds while eating nuts, but suddenly their bodies develop sensitivity, and the nuts begin to stall the weight loss. This is an example of why tracking your food and listening to your body is so important.

Take Charge of the Meal at Restaurants and Stay on Track

When reviewing a restaurant menu, the first step is to identify potential hidden sugars in various dishes. Sugar can appear in many forms, including syrups, sauces, and even dressings. Look out for items that contain words such as sweetened," "glazed," or "marinade," as these often indicate added sugar. Be cautious of healthy options, such as fruit juices. or smoothies, which can also be laden with hidden sugars. Familiarizing yourself with common aliases for sugar, such as sucrose, fructose, or high-fructose corn syrup, can help you make more informed choices. Next, focus on the foundational elements of a meal: proteins, vegetables, and healthy fats. Most menus will offer a variety of options, such as grilled meats, seafood, or plant-based proteins like tofu. Opt for dishes that are prepared with minimal sauces or dressings, as these can often contain added sugar.

You may be surprised to know that salads are usually not the best choice because you have no way of knowing how much protein and fat you are getting. Vegetables not only enhance the nutritional value of your meal but also provide satisfying flavors without sugar. Don't be afraid to customize your order. Be aggressive with your server if necessary. These days, restaurants are willing to accommodate dietary preferences, especially when it comes to making a dish sugar-free. You can request alterations such as omitting sauces, substituting sides, or asking for grilled instead of fried items. This not only ensures you enjoy a meal that aligns with your dietary goals but also empowers you to take control of your food choices. Being assertive about your needs can lead to a more enjoyable dining experience and can often inspire restaurants to offer more sugar-free options in the future.

When to Eat Carbs

Think of carbs like a knob on a radio dial. Turn the volume down (on low for a while) while you are giving your body the time it needs to release fat. Turn up the volume slightly when you feel strong enough to add in a carb or cheat meal. Adjust your dial based on how you are feeling, how your stomach is feeling, and how quickly you want to lose on the scale.

Tip: The more carbs you have each week the slower your weight loss will be. But this does not mean you cannot have them. Plan them in, be. strategic, and make sure it is 100% worth it in that moment. I have found that most people who are overweight think they can never eat carbs. If you feel you gain weight quickly, especially in the belly area, this is a sign that one of your root causes is insulin resistance. This means that what you have been eating has been spiking your blood sugar levels for too often and too long. Your body has become insulin-resistant (too many glucose spikes). Do a sugar detox for 10 days. Then, rebuild your nutrition habits to stabilize your blood sugar levels.

Over time, you can add the "good carbs" back in slowly and in small portions. Yes. It will require some sacrifice until you reach that point, depending on how much you would like to lose, but it is not about eating low carb forever. Be patient with yourself and do the work that is necessary now, so that you enjoy the carbs later.

TIP: When we have excess weight on the body, carbs (which turn to sugar in the body) make it easy for the body to store fat. Choose to avoid them for now and give your body the time it needs to heal. The carbs will be back in when your body is ready to manage them. Your body will not be as reactive to carbs forever if you do the work now.

TIP: When the time is right, start adding small portions of good complex carbohydrates (nature's carbs) Complex carbohydrates (potatoes, beans root vegetables, bananas, fruits).

Fruits and Weight Loss

Fruits are healthy, but they are still sugar. Depending on where you are in your weight loss journey, I would suggest sticking with apples berries, and grapefruit for the first 3-5 weeks or until you are certain you are not feeling tempted by the taste of sugar. The juicy fruits (watermelon, grapes, mangos) should be added back in at the back end of your journey because they significantly impact blood sugar in post-people. Give your body a chance to release weight then add them once or twice a week until you are at your goal weight.

TIP Bannas are the worst for weight loss. It is best to avoid them.

When Clean Eating Does Not Produce Weight Loss

When we eat whole food nutrition, we are basically "eating clean." While it is important to eat clean when it comes to weight loss, sometimes that is not enough. The body becomes resistant and, in some cases, the weight loss just stalls. Why does this happen?

Eating clean food for some people may mean that although they are eating healthy foods, their portion sizes are out of balance and not signaling weight loss in the body.

9 Root Causes of Weight Loss Stalls when you are eating clean or on a plant-based nutrition plan.

Eating vegetables and low protein.

Having too many smoothies containing fruit

Mainly eating fruit and no vegetables

Eating too many starchy vegetables (causing elevated blood sugar spikes.

Too many Juicy fruits are higher glycemic and keep the body in a state of elevated blood sugar.

Not eating enough quality protein.

Not eating enough healthy fat.

Not enough calories.

TIP 1: Track your food for 7 days. Minimize the juicy fruits and replace them with apples or berries.

TIP 2: Increase protein with fish or chicken.

TIP 3: If you are eating processed plant-based protein products- (burgers or vegan products) replace them with tofu.

PUFAS (Vegetable Oils) – Major Root Cause of Yo-Yo Rebound Weight Gain

What are PUFA's? (Polyunsaturated Fats) are fatty acids in seed oils.

Corn Oil

Cottonseed Oil

Soybean Oil

Soy

Canola Oil

Sunflower

Rice Bran – typically used in restaurants.

Grapeseed Oil – typically used in restaurants.

What is the Impact of Vegetable Oils on Our Body

These seed oils are what make junk food junk, and they shorten our lifespan.

A. Vegetable oils make our food toxic.

B. They make our body fat toxic because they reformulate our body fat with polyunsaturated fatty acids far more than the human body has ever had before in the industrial era. These toxins in our visceral fat are why visceral fat (fat around our organs) is so dangerous to our health.

C. Vegetable oils make our food toxic.

D. They make our body fat toxic because they reformulate our body fat with polyunsaturated fatty acids far more than the human body has ever had before in the industrial era.

E. These toxins in our visceral fat are why visceral fat (fat around our organs) is so dangerous to our health.

It is important to understand what **your** body fat is. Body fat is an organ that is supposed to have a positive role in our body- just like the other organs in our body. You may have not heard about body fat addressed in this way, but it is supposed to be our ally, as an independent organ, and its role is to be able to fuel your cells with energy *between* meals.

When vegetable oils are in our diets, we build body fat that our cells do not want to burn off. In other words, we can build body fat but cannot get rid of it easily. The other issue is the cumulative effect. Many of us grew up eating this oil and the damage was done to our metabolism.

When the main source of our dietary fat is seed oils. They are chemically different than the fats we used to eat. Their fatty acid makeup is different, and they are high in PUFA's. As a result, our body fat becomes vastly different which means that body fat can no longer do its job of supplying energy between meals.

The heat, chemicals, and treatment that happens in the industrial factory damage the oil and create toxins that are then distributed throughout our bodies. Seed oils turn body fat into a toxic generating machine. These oils are commonly used in our everyday products including high-end minimally processed foods. The oils have been linked to obesity, heart disease, diabetes, and brain conditions.

Superfood

Incorporating superfoods into your diet can help support weight loss and overall health. Superfoods are nutrient-dense foods that provide a wide range of health benefits including helping you to slim down. o slim down and stay strong.

One particularly beneficial superfood is salmon. This fatty fish is rich in omega-3 fatty acids, which have been shown to reduce inflammation, improve heart health, and support weight loss. In addition, salmon is a great source of protein, which can help keep you full and satisfied, making it easier to stick to a healthy diet. Try incorporating salmon into your meals at least twice a week to reap the benefits.

Another superfood that you should consider adding to your plan is kale. This leafy green vegetable is packed with vitamins, minerals, and antioxidants that can help support weight loss and overall health. Kale is also low in calories and high in fiber. Try adding kale to salads, smoothies, or stir-fries to boost your nutrient intake and support your weight loss goals.

Berries are another superfood that can benefit anyone who wants to lose weight. Berries are rich in antioxidants, fiber, and vitamins, making them a great choice for a healthy snack or dessert. They are low glycemic and low calorie, making them a great option to satisfy your sweet tooth without derailing your weight loss efforts. Try incorporating a variety of berries like blueberries, strawberries, and raspberries into your diet regularly to support your weight loss goals. In addition to salmon, kale, and berries, there are many other superfood examples including avocados, quinoa, and chia seeds, all of which are nutrient-dense foods that can help support weight loss and overall health.

CHAPTER 5:
How Sugar Affects Weight Loss

The Different Types of Sugar

Sugar is a common ingredient in many diets, and understanding its distinct types can significantly influence weight management. This subchapter delves into the diverse types of sugar, shedding light on their distinct characteristics and how they affect the body, particularly in the context of weight gain. As women often face unique metabolic and hormonal challenges, recognizing the nuances of sugar can empower informed dietary choices.

The most recognized type of sugar is sucrose, commonly known as table sugar. Sucrose is a disaccharide composed of glucose and fructose and is found naturally in many plants, particularly in sugarcane and sugar beets. In moderation, sucrose can be part of a balanced diet, but excessive consumption is linked to weight gain and other health issues. Women, who may experience fluctuating hormone levels, can find that even small increases in sucrose intake can lead to cravings and increased appetite, making it essential to monitor its presence in everyday foods. When looking at food labels- look for anything ending in "ose" and avoid them Another important type of sugar is fructose, a monosaccharide found in fruits, honey, and root vegetables. While naturally occurring, fructose

is healthier, the rise of high-fructose corn syrup (HFCS) in processed foods acts as a poison in the e body. HFCS is often found in sugary beverages and snacks, contributing to higher calorie intake without providing the satiety that whole foods offer. For women aiming to lose weight, it is crucial to differentiate between the beneficial effects of natural fructose from whole fruits and the detrimental effects of added sugars like HFCS, which can lead to increased fat accumulation and the development of diabetes and heart disease.

Glucose, another monosaccharide, plays a vital role in the body's energy supply. It is rapidly absorbed into the bloodstream, causing a quick rise in blood sugar levels. This spike can lead to a subsequent crash, prompting the body to crave more sugar for a quick energy boost. Women, who may experience more pronounced blood sugar fluctuations due to hormonal changes, should be mindful of their glucose intake. Foods high in refined carbohydrates often lead to rapid glucose spikes, which can trigger overeating and weight gain.

Lastly, there's lactose, the sugar found in milk and dairy products. While lactose is less of a concern for many individuals, those with lactose intolerance may struggle with its consumption. Dairy can be a source of essential nutrients, yet many of us find that full-fat dairy products can contribute to our weight gain when consumed in excess. Understanding how different sugars interact within the body and affect cravings and metabolism can help women make better choices regarding dairy and other sugar sources.

NATURAL SWEETENERS

Monk Fruit- -Agave-Honey-Coconut Sugar -Maple Syrup -Stevia- Fructose, Fruit Sugar

Sugar is sugar. When it comes to weight loss, less is best, but the overall goal is to choose the sugars that have the least impact on your blood sugar levels.

First Choice- Stevia Leaf

Better Choice – Fruit sugars(fructose)

Good choice- Raw Honey. Local honey is best.

Sugar Addiction

Signs and symptoms tell you that your body is addicted to sugar. Brain fog

- Sugar cravings
- Bloating,

- Headaches
- Afternoon sluggishness
- Nighttime cravings for sugar
- You never feel full.

Sugar addiction leads to the occurrence of mood swings and variations in energy levels. The rapid spikes, (blood sugar rollercoaster) and subsequent crashes in blood sugar levels, caused by frequent and high sugar intake, lead to irritability, fatigue, and difficulties in maintaining stable emotional well-being. It is also common to be addicted to sugar and not realize it. This means that they are not necessarily craving sugary foods, but that the body itself is addicted to sugar. The sugars can come from natural sugars such as fruit, potatoes, bread or sweets, and desserts.

How Sugar Affects the Body

Sugar, a ubiquitous ingredient in many diets, plays a significant role in weight gain and overall health. When consumed, sugar quickly absorbs into the bloodstream, leading to a rapid increase in blood glucose levels. This spike triggers the pancreas to release insulin, a hormone that helps cells absorb glucose for energy. However, excessive sugar consumption can overwhelm this system, resulting in elevated insulin levels. High insulin levels not only promote fat storage but also inhibit the body's ability to use fat as a source of energy. For women, who may already face hormonal fluctuations throughout their lives, managing insulin levels becomes crucial in preventing unwanted weight gain.

The type of sugar consumed also matters greatly. Depending on sugar, the impacts on blood sugar are different for each of us. Simple sugars, found in processed foods and sugary beverages, are rapidly digested and provide a quick energy boost. However, this rapid digestion can lead to a subsequent crash in energy levels, prompting more cravings and potentially leading to overeating. In contrast, complex carbohydrates, which contain fiber, digest more slowly, providing sustained energy and reducing the likelihood of spikes and crashes.

Sugar also impacts mood and mental health and is closely tied to eating behaviors. Research has shown that high sugar intake may contribute to feelings of anxiety and depression. Emotional eating can become a coping mechanism, leading to a cycle of consuming sugary foods to boost mood, followed by guilt and further weight gain. Understanding this relationship between sugar, mood, and eating habits is vital for women seeking to navigate their weight loss journey effectively. Developing healthier coping strategies and making mindful choices about sugar intake can help break this cycle.

Additionally, excessive sugar consumption has been linked to inflammation in the body. Chronic inflammation can disrupt hormonal balance, affecting metabolism and leading to increased fat storage.

If you are overweight and have health conditions you are particularly susceptible to the effects of inflammation, as it can exacerbate conditions like polycystic ovary syndrome (PCOS) and hormonal imbalances that affect weight. By reducing sugar intake and opting for anti-inflammatory foods, you can support the body in maintaining a healthy weight and overall well-being.

Sugar's Impact on Appetite Regulation

Sugar's impact on appetite regulation is a crucial aspect to consider. If you typically choose to satisfy sugar cravings with "sugar-free" or sweets that use sugar alcohol they may be influencing how sugar influences your hunger signals and satiety. When sugar is consumed, (any form of sweetness that you can taste on your tongue) it triggers a series of hormonal responses in the body that can alter appetite regulation. Specifically, sugars can lead to spikes in insulin levels, which in turn can affect the hormone leptin—responsible for signaling fullness—resulting in increased feelings of hunger soon after consumption.

TIP: When you have uncontrollable sugar cravings for something decadent and you feel powerless to avoid it- use sugar-free snacks as your way through that moment. Use them as a tool to help you minimize the damage of calorie excess in sugar binges or emotional eating moments.

The immediate effects of sugar on the body can create a cycle of cravings and overeating. When high-sugar foods are consumed, they lead to a rapid increase in blood glucose levels, providing a quick source of energy. However, this spike is often followed by a crash, as insulin is released to manage the excess sugar in the bloodstream. This fluctuation can leave women feeling fatigued and craving more sugar or carbohydrates to regain that energy, perpetuating a cycle that undermines weight loss efforts.

Sugar also affects the brain's reward system, causing dopamine spikes (feel-good hormones) making sweet foods more appealing and reinforcing the desire to consume them. Research has shown that the consumption of sugar can activate the same pleasure centers in the brain that are triggered by addictive substances. This response can lead to a preference for sugary foods over healthier options, further complicating appetite regulation. As you navigate your dietary choices, recognizing this behavioral aspect of sugar consumption is essential in breaking free from the cycle of dependence on sweet foods.

In addition to immediate appetite changes, long-term sugar consumption can lead to metabolic alterations that affect how the body processes food. High sugar intake has been linked to an increased risk of developing insulin resistance, a condition where the body's cells become less responsive to insulin. This can create a feedback loop that not only disrupts hunger signals but also promotes fat storage, making weight loss increasingly challenging. Understanding these metabolic consequences can empower you to make strategic choices about sugar intake that support your weight loss goals.

How Sugar Feeds Your Emotional Eating Patterns

Emotional eating is a common phenomenon that many of you are struggling with. Eating episodes and binges are often in response to stress, anxiety, or other emotional triggers. When faced with uncomfortable feelings, some may turn to food, particularly sugary treats, as a source of comfort. This behavior can create a cycle where emotional states drive consumption, leading to weight gain and further emotional distress. Understanding the link between emotions and sugar cravings is crucial for people who want to build a healthy relationship with food.

Sugar plays a significant role in emotional eating due to its ability to provide quick energy and instant gratification. When consumed, sugar stimulates the release of neurotransmitters like dopamine, which can enhance mood temporarily. This pleasurable response can lead to the addictive need to seek out sugary foods during times of stress or sadness. The immediate gratification and feeling good response mistakenly intensify the belief that these foods will alleviate their emotional discomfort. Unfortunately, this immediate relief is often followed by a crash in energy levels and mood, perpetuating a vicious cycle of emotional eating that can contribute to weight gain.

In moments of emotional turmoil, sugary foods can seem like a refuge. This is referred to as "eating your feelings" or "stuffing" your feelings. It provides a momentary escape and a way to be distracted from the actual root source of emotions. However, this coping mechanism can have detrimental effects on both physical and emotional health, as excess sugar intake is linked to weight gain, increased cravings, and even long-term health issues such as diabetes and heart disease.

TIP: Journal the things you eat that are a result of emotional or binge eating. Keep track of what the catalysts are that are causing the eating event(s) to happen. Was it related to work stress, fighting with your spouse, or sadness? Whatever it is, track your emotions and the corresponding food choices to identify your triggers.

To break the cycle of emotional eating and reduce sugar consumption, it is important to develop healthier coping strategies. Mindful eating practices can help you become more aware of your hunger cues and emotional triggers, allowing you to make more conscious food choices. Additionally, finding alternative ways to cope with stress—such as exercise, meditation, or engaging in hobbies—can help diminish the reliance on sugar-laden comfort foods. By cultivating a supportive environment and establishing a routine that prioritizes emotional well--

being, it is easier to be consistent with healthier habits that promote weight loss and overall health.

TIP: One of the root causes of emotional eating is sugar addiction.

SUGAR ALCOHOLS

Check your ingredient labels for chemicals and sugar alcohol that spike your blood sugar. Food manufacturers are not held to any type of accountability for false labeling. Example: Just because a keto product says that it is low carb does not mean that the product is going to help you lose weight. It will still spike your glucose levels. There are over sixty chemical names for sugar. The front of a label may state that it does not contain sugar, or "no sugar added"- but the ingredient label tells you the real story. Chemical sugars in the ingredient label are not factored into their analysis and will significantly affect your blood sugar levels and slow down your weight loss.

Recognizing Symptoms of Leptin Resistance

Recognizing the signs and symptoms of leptin resistance is crucial to reclaiming optimal metabolic health. Leptin, often referred to as the "satiety hormone," plays a vital role in regulating energy balance and body weight.

When the body becomes resistant to leptin, its ability to signal fullness diminishes, which can lead to overeating and weight gain. Understanding the common indicators of leptin resistance can empower you to take initiative-taking steps toward achieving your wellness goals.

One of the most prevalent signs of leptin resistance is persistent hunger, even after eating adequate amounts of food. If you are experiencing this symptom, you may find yourself reaching for snacks shortly after meals, feeling unsatisfied despite consuming calorie-dense foods. This relentless urge to eat can stem from the brain's inability to recognize leptin signals, leading to a cycle of overeating and further metabolic disruption. Recognizing this symptom is the first step toward addressing underlying hormonal imbalances. Another common symptom is difficulty losing weight or maintaining weight loss, despite efforts in diet and exercise. This can be attributed to the body's altered response to leptin, which affects metabolism and fat storage. It is essential to understand that the scale is not the only measure of progress; improving metabolic health can manifest in other ways, such as increased energy levels and enhanced overall well-being.

Fatigue and low energy levels are also significant indicators of leptin resistance. Women may experience a constant feeling of tiredness, which can be exacerbated by poor sleep quality often associated with hormonal imbalances. When leptin signaling is disrupted, the body may struggle to regulate energy levels efficiently, leading to a sense of lethargy. Addressing leptin resistance can help restore energy balance, allowing women to feel revitalized and more capable of engaging in physical activity.

Don't Eat After 6:00 pm

Eating at night or going to bed on a full stomach starts the process of leptin resistance. It causes your hormones to go haywire and your metabolism stops any fat burning. It will also trigger cortisol spikes (stress hormones), heartburn, low melatonin, poor sleep, insomnia, and thyroid issues. Your thyroid regulates metabolism and is most active when you are sleeping. Our body wants to be repaired and restored overnight. If it has work to do with digesting and assimilating food during that time, the potential for weight gain increases. If you are experiencing symptoms such as sugar cravings, or never feeling full, chances are good that your leptin signaling is out of balance and it is a contributing source to weight gain.

CHAPTER 6.
Big Food and Big Pharma

Do They Deserve Our Trust?

If you search on Google for weight loss, there are dozens of ways to lose weight and most of them do not focus on how to keep the weight off Adding to the confusion are the big food companies taking advantage of how intensely people want to lose weight. Do not be a victim of false claims and advertising. I want to help you take a closer look into the root cause of why and how food manufacturing companies are impacting the obesity rates today.

When we look at Big Food and Big Pharma from a commonsense perspective, they are business. They profit and make money when we are sick and fat. Every year, more "breakthrough pharmaceuticals" and "organic healthy products" come out on the market, yet as a country, we have only gotten sicker and fatter, and the obesity epidemic has skyrocketed.

If you have dieted throughout your life and tried one or more of the national diet programs, (Jenny Craig, Weight Watchers, Nutrisystem) you may have already gained the weight back plus additional pounds. Why does this happen? I can tell you it is not because you lack willpower or discipline. Those programs are effective for weight loss, but what is the common denominator in all of them? They do not teach you how to maintain and sustain a healthy lifestyle that feels good and adapted to your lifestyle. They are also too expensive to do on a long-term basis. A few of them offer "weight loss food" which is just more processed food. They are feeding the obesity epidemic in the US.

Keto is the latest diet that can be highly effective for weight loss, but I have found many people stop losing on keto- partly because many people incorporate keto products or gluten-free products. Although the products are low carb, the ingredients added by the manufacturer have a far worse impact on the body than carbohydrates.

American Diabetes Association

The American Diabetes Association was founded in 1939 by six physicians. Dr. Herman O Mosenthal, Dr. Joseph T. Beard Wood Jr, Dr. Joseph H. Barach, and Dr. E. S. Dillion. These doctors had nothing but the best of intentions to help people. But over time, things have changed, and the guidelines that the ADA advises for people with diabetes are wrong. In early 2000 the ADA struck a three-year, $1.5 million sponsorship deal with Cadbury- Schweppes, the world's largest confectioner product including Diet-Rite soda, Snapple, unsweetened tea, and Motts Apple Juice- who benefits from this scenario?

All forms of diabetes can be reversed. The average doctor does not know what to tell their patients with diabetes and as a result, refers their patients for diet guidance to the American Diabetes Association.

Facts To Know About the ADA to Further Investigate

Recipes posted on the ADA website that will make diabetes worse. Most of them are either low nutrient-dense or have added sugars (hidden sugars). The question becomes, why would they encourage people with diabetes to eat meals that would ensure that their blood sugar levels remain high?

The ADA accepts millions of dollars every year, from the manufacturers of insulin and other diabetes medications, and they accept millions of dollars in "donations" from Big Food companies and Big Pharma. Who benefits from this- the companies or us as the consumer?

How To Reverse Diabetes and Lose Weight

As a naturopathic doctor practicing for the last 13 years, I have helped hundreds of patients reverse their conditions with nutrition adjustments.

Medications can typically be eliminated unless it is an end-stage condition. If you have any form of diabetes, please reach out to a nutritionist or trusted healthcare provider who understands how to apply nutrition to stabilize blood sugar levels naturally. Diabetes can be reversed in as little as 30 days with a personalized approach to stabilize your unique glucose levels.

The following are the guidelines that I give my patients as we work on weight loss and reversing diabetes. If your doctor has different guidelines for you and your diabetes is not improving, take this list to your doctor to open the discussion. Their goal should be to get you off medications.

1. Minimize whole grains.
2. Eat more healthy fat.
3. Avoid oat oatmeal. It has a major impact on blood sugar levels for most people.
4. Wear a glucose monitor for 30 days straight to assess all the foods you eat.

Do not eat carbs in moderation- minimize them as much as possible. All carbs turn to sugar upon digestion which will elevate blood sugar. The ADA recommends oatmeal as a staple breakfast

Do not add a sugar source of any kind to manage dizziness, hypoglycemia, or lightheadedness. Eat a protein snack instead. (hard-boiled egg or string cheese

Eat more protein, not less.

Your A1c goal should be less than 5.2. (Not 5.7 – 6-2).

TIP: Ask your doctor what his/her long-term goal is for you. Is it to get off all insulin and medications and reverse the condition?

How to Maximize Your Weight Loss Each Week

- Eat a savory protein breakfast in the morning. Build your breakfast around protein (eggs, yogurt, nuts, quality protein powder and add healthy fat and fiber) If you want something sweet and low in sugar, eat apples or berries.

- Avoid sweet breakfasts. The big food companies started us down that path 20 years ago with cereals, breakfast bars, cakes, and pies. If you begin your day with a carb/ sugar breakfast, you jump onto the early morning ride on the blood sugar rollercoaster.

- Take Apple Cider Vinegar (liquid not gummies.. Vinegar has many proven weight loss benefits. The acetic acid in vinegar temporarily inactivates alpha-amylase as a result, sugar and starch are transformed into glucose more slowly, and the glucose hits our system more softly- lessening the impact of the spike.

- Move after eating a meal. The immediate calorie burning will reduce cortisol and blood sugar levels.

- Wait at least 3 hours between all meals or snacks It takes three hours for your body to complete digestion. If you eat too soon it will significantly spike your glucose levels and slow down weight loss for that day.

Meal Planning Tips

Meal planning is an essential aspect of your weight loss journey. By taking the time to plan out your meals in advance, you can ensure that you are making healthy choices and staying on track with your goals. Here are some meal planning tips to help you achieve your weight loss goals. When planning your meals, include a variety of foods to ensure you are getting a wide range of nutrients. Each meal should include plenty of fruit and vegetables, lean proteins, and healthy fats. Experiment with different recipes to keep things interesting and prevent meal boredom. Some women find meal planning very overwhelming because it is one more thing on their "to-do" list, but this is a habit worth making a priority. It is an excellent way to help restore the feeling of being in control. If you have meals ready to go, the day will run much smoother. Plus, you will feel better and have more energy because you are fueling your body properly.

Complex carbs should be eaten sparingly if the goal is weight loss. Examples of good carbohydrates include beans, sweet potatoes, corn, quinoa, fruits, and oats. Although they are healthy, they still cause spikes in most people and should be eaten in small portions. Learn to listen to your body's signals when you are eating a meal. If you are suddenly feeling bloated during a meal, this is a sign that something you are eating is rapidly elevating your blood sugar levels. Another important tip for successful meal planning is to set aside time each week to plan out your meals and create a shopping list. By taking the time to plan, you can avoid the temptation to grab unhealthy convenience foods when you are short on time. Make a list of the ingredients you will need for each meal and stick to it when you go grocery shopping.

In addition to planning out your meals, it is also important to have healthy snacks on hand to prevent mindless munching on unhealthy foods. Keep a variety of nutritious snacks like nuts, seeds, string cheese, or Greek yogurt in your pantry or refrigerator. By having healthy options readily available, you can avoid reaching for sugary or high-calorie snacks and chips.

Don't be afraid to seek support and accountability in your meal-planning journey. Consider joining a weight loss support group, enlisting the help of a friend or family member, or working with a health coach to help you stay on track with your goals. Having someone to share your successes and struggles with can make an enormous difference in your weight loss journey. If you do not have access to a group program but feel comfortable working virtually, please reach out to me. All my weight loss plans at DrLoriMahler.com include weight loss counseling.

Water Intake - How Much is Enough?

Most of us realize the importance of drinking water but find it hard to drink enough throughout the day. Combining hydration with nutrition is a vital aspect of achieving optimal metabolic function and effective weight management. Water plays a crucial role in numerous bodily processes, including digestion, nutrient absorption, and the regulation of body temperature. When we consider how hydration interacts with the food we eat, it becomes evident that the two are inextricably linked. Proper hydration not only enhances metabolism but also aids in the efficient breakdown of macronutrients, ensuring that you can maximize the benefits of your diet while promoting fat loss. The relationship between water and metabolism cannot be overstated.

Studies have shown that adequate hydration can increase metabolic rates, with some research suggesting that drinking cold water can elevate energy expenditure as the body works to heat the water to body temperature. For women, this means that incorporating sufficient water intake throughout the day can serve as a simple yet effective strategy for boosting metabolism. Additionally, hydration plays a crucial role in the breakdown of carbohydrates, fats, and proteins. When your body is well-hydrated, it can efficiently process these macronutrients, leading to improved energy levels and reduced cravings, both of which are essential for weight management.

Nutrition and hydration also work hand in hand to optimize performance and recovery. If you are engaged in regular physical activity, staying hydrated is essential for maintaining endurance and strength. Dehydration can lead to fatigue, decreased coordination, and impaired recovery, all of which can hinder your fitness goals. By combining the right hydration strategies with a balanced diet rich in vitamins, minerals, and other nutrients, you can enhance your overall energy levels and performance. This synergy not only supports weight loss but also promotes a healthier lifestyle, fostering a positive relationship with food and exercise.

The timing of hydration to meals can significantly impact weight management. Drinking water before meals can help control appetite, leading to reduced overall caloric intake. This practice not only aids in portion control but also enhances digestion. When you are adequately hydrated before eating, the digestive system functions more efficiently, allowing for better absorption of nutrients. This means that every meal becomes an opportunity to nourish the body while also supporting hydration needs, creating a holistic approach to health and wellness.

Lastly, choosing hydrating foods can further enhance the benefits of combining hydration with nutrition. Many fruits and vegetables, such as cucumbers, watermelon, and oranges, have high water content and provide essential nutrients. Incorporating these foods into your daily meals can help you stay hydrated while also delivering vital vitamins and minerals that support metabolic health. By understanding the interconnectedness of hydration and nutrition, women can adopt a more comprehensive strategy that not only aids in fat loss but promotes overall well-being, making it a cornerstone of their health journey.

Tip: You should be drinking half of your total body weight in ounces each day. Are you drinking enough?

CHAPTER 7:
Exercise and Fitness

Exercise is a key component in achieving weight loss and maintaining a healthy lifestyle. Regular physical activity not only helps in shedding those extra pounds but also improves overall health and well-being. One of the key benefits of exercise is its ability to boost metabolism. As we age the metabolism tends to slow down, but we can compensate and assist our body with fat burning by engaging in regular physical activity, such as strength training and cardio. Regular physical activity and resistance training can help in lowering blood pressure, improving cholesterol levels, and maintaining bone density. It also has been linked to improved mental health, reduced stress levels, and better sleep quality.

Exercise has hundreds of benefits, but it is also important to be strategic about adding it to your daily habits. If you dread or hate working out it will only make your journey, feel harder and impossible to attain. Sustainable weight loss will come through your nutrition and what you put into your body. Start with the food changes as 90% of your effort. All your motivation, willpower, and money need to go towards eating the

TIP: If you are trying to lose weight and have not or do not like to exercise, consider starting a routine after you are feeling confident about your new nutritional habits. This approach works extremely well for my clients who hate to exercise. Your goal should be Nutrition first, and exercise second.

As we age, our bodies undergo various changes that can make it more challenging to maintain a healthy weight and stay physically active. Incorporating regular exercise into a weekly routine will help you build a healthy, streamlined body composition. In this subchapter, we will explore the different types of exercises that are particularly effective for weight loss.

Cardiovascular exercise helps to improve heart health, increase endurance, and burn calories. Add in variety such as activities brisk walking, jogging, cycling, swimming, or aerobics in their routine. As you plan your workouts each week, keep in mind that too much cardio will slow down your weight loss progress.

Strength training should be an essential component when trying to lose weight. Consider adding some sort of weight resistance during every workout to ensure the stimulation of muscle growth. Setting a goal to take a brisk walk after dinner for longer than 15 minutes should include an additional 10-15 strength training session. This will boost your metabolism and increase your overall strength and stamina. Some examples of effective strength training exercises include squats, lunges, push-ups, and bicep curls.

Flexibility and balance exercises are also beneficial because they can help improve mobility, prevent injuries, and enhance overall quality of life. Yoga, Pilates, and tai chi are great options for improving flexibility, balance, and core strength. These types of exercises can also help alleviate stress and promote relaxation, which is important for overall well-being. Be sure to incorporate the activities you enjoy and fit with your lifestyle. Whether it is dancing, hiking, swimming, or playing a sport, finding activities that bring joy, and satisfaction can help you stay motivated and committed to your exercise routine. Remember to listen to your body, start slowly and gradually increase the intensity and duration of your workouts as you become stronger and more confident.

By incorporating a variety of exercises into your routine, you can improve your overall health, boost your metabolism, support weight loss, and enhance your quality of life. Consistency is key, so make exercise a priority in your daily routine and reap the many benefits that come with staying active and fit.

Creating a Workout Routine

The goal is to create a workout routine that you feel is challenging enough to get you results but also that you enjoy. If you have serious goals and want to achieve weight loss and maintain overall health, it is important to consider your fitness level and any physical limitations you may have. Consult with a healthcare provider or fitness professional before starting any new exercise program to ensure it is safe and effective for your individual needs.

When designing your workout routine, consider scheduling your workouts at a time that is convenient for you and fits into your daily routine. This could be first thing in the morning, during your lunch break, or in the evening after work. It is important to find a time that works best for you to help you develop a consistent schedule that ensures you stay on track with your fitness goals. Choose workouts that will fuel your motivation, burn fat, and make you feel powerful.

When Is the Best Time to Exercise

Should you exercise before a meal? Not necessarily. Exercising after meals seems to be the best option, but before is also useful. There was a study done on resistance training for obese people. They exercised before dinner (eating 30 minutes after the workout was over). It lowered their glucose and insulin spikes by 18 percent and 35 percent, respectively, as opposed to 30 percent and 48 percent if the exercise was started 45 minutes after dinner.

Exercising anytime is fantastic, and it has many more positive side effects than just curbing a glucose spike. Among other things, it helps increase your mental well-being, energizes us, reduces inflammation, and helps to reset your gut microbiome. You will lose weight faster if your gut is digesting food properly.

Mindset and Motivation

Overcoming Mental Blocks

Mental blocks are one of the biggest obstacles that we face when trying to lose weight. These mental barriers can prevent us from reaching our weight loss goals and can make the journey feel impossible. However, it is important to recognize that you can overcome mental blocks with the right mindset and strategies.

TIP: Example of a mental block. Feeling as though you cannot get past a certain number on the scale. Believe that you will break through it.

The first step in overcoming mental blocks is to identify what is holding you back. Are you afraid of failure? Do you have negative thoughts about your ability to lose weight? Do you believe that you CAN reach your goal? By acknowledging these thoughts and feelings, you can begin to work through them and develop a plan to overcome them.

One effective strategy for overcoming mental blocks is to focus on the positive aspects of weight loss and the benefits it will bring to your life. Instead of dwelling on the challenges and obstacles, try to shift your mindset to focus on the rewards that come with achieving your weight loss goals. Visualize how you will feel when you reach your target weight and what your life will look like when you reach your goal.

Another helpful strategy is to surround yourself with a supportive community of like-minded individuals who are also on a weight loss journey. This can provide you with encouragement, accountability, and motivation to keep pushing forward. By sharing your struggles and successes with others, you can gain valuable insights and support that can help you overcome mental blocks.

Overcoming mental blocks is a crucial step in achieving weight loss success. By identifying and being aware of your mental barriers, focusing on the positive aspects of weight loss, and surrounding yourself with a supportive community, you can overcome these obstacles and reach your weight loss goals. You have the power to change your mindset and overcome any mental blocks that may be holding you back from achieving the slim and strong body you desire.

Staying Motivated

Staying motivated on your weight loss journey can be challenging. However, with the right mindset and strategies, you can stay on track and achieve your goals. In this chapter, we will explore some tips and tricks to help you stay motivated and focused on your weight loss journey.

One of the best ways to stay motivated is to set realistic and achievable goals. Instead of aiming for a drastic weight loss in a short period of time, focus on setting small, achievable goals that you can reach each week or month. Celebrate your successes along the way and use them as motivation to keep going.

Another crucial factor in staying motivated is finding a support system. Surround yourself with friends, family, or even a weight loss group who can cheer you on and hold you accountable. Having someone to share your successes and struggles with can make a significant difference in staying motivated and on track.

Lastly, remember to be kind to yourself and practice self-care. Weight loss can be a challenging journey! It is important to take care of yourself both physically and mentally. Treat yourself with compassion and kindness and remember that progress takes time. By staying motivated and focused on your goals, you can achieve the slim and strong body that you desire.

Self-Care – Place Yourself on Your Priority List

Too often, I see clients avoiding important self-care practices that are essential for maintaining overall health and achieving weight loss. Taking care of yourself both physically and mentally can have a significant impact on your weight loss journey. In this subchapter, we will explore some self-care practices that can help you achieve your weight loss goals and improve your overall quality of life.

One important self-care practice is to get enough sleep. I am sure this is a huge problem for many of you. Lack of sleep can disrupt your body's hormones and metabolism, making it harder to lose weight. Aim for 7-9 hours of quality sleep each night to help support your weight loss efforts. Creating a bedtime ritual and practicing relaxation techniques before bed can help you get a better night's sleep.

Another self-care practice to prioritize is stress management. Chronic stress can lead to weight gain and make it difficult to lose weight. Finding healthy ways to manage stress, such as meditation, yoga, or deep breathing exercises, can help you stay on track with your weight loss goals. It is important to take time for yourself each day to relax and unwind, whether it's through exercise, spending time in nature, or enjoying a hobby you love.

Remember to listen to your body, take time for yourself, and make self-care a priority in your daily routine. You are worth the time, and effort and deserve to feel happy and healthy in your body.

CHAPTER 8:
Break Sugar Addiction

The Science Behind Cravings

The phenomenon of cravings is a complex interplay of biological, psychological, and environmental factors that often become more pronounced with age. As you navigate changes in metabolism, hormonal fluctuations, and emotional health, understanding the science behind cravings becomes essential. Cravings can manifest as an intense desire for specific foods or substances, and they can significantly impact your weight loss efforts. Delving into the underlying mechanisms of cravings will help you identify triggers and specific foods that may be signaling the imbalances in your body that need attention.

Cravings can feel different to each of us. You may crave sugar, salt, or savory foods. Although many of us struggle with sugar cravings, both salt and sugar cravings can be a signal that your body is deficient in one or more nutrients. Learning to tune in and "listen" to your body. It is always speaking to you.

At a biological level, cravings are influenced by neurotransmitters, hormones, and the body's energy balance. Dopamine, often referred to as the "feel-good" neurotransmitter, plays a crucial role in the reward stem of the brain. When we consume foods that are high in sugar or fat, dopamine is released, creating a sense of pleasure, and reinforcing the desire for those foods. As we age, dopamine levels may fluctuate, making us more susceptible to cravings for calorie-dense foods that provide quick energy and satisfaction. Understanding this connection can help you recognize the triggers behind their cravings.

Hormonal changes, particularly those associated with menopause in women and andropause in men, can further exacerbate cravings. For many, these transitions can lead to mood swings, increased stress, and feelings of anxiety, all of which can drive cravings for comfort foods. The body's natural response to stress often involves seeking out high-sugar or high-fat foods as a form of emotional regulation. By acknowledging these hormonal shifts and their impact on cravings, individuals can adopt mindful practices and aromatherapy techniques to soothe emotional distress, reducing the likelihood of turning to unhealthy food choices.

Emotional and psychological triggers play a significant role in our cravings and overall well-being, particularly as we age. For those over 40, understanding these triggers becomes essential for maintaining a balanced weight and lifestyle. I have seen many of my patients encounter various stressors, such as career changes, family dynamics, and health concerns. Those types of factors can lead you down the path to emotional eating or cravings for unhealthy substances, making it imperative to recognize the underlying emotional states that fuel these desires.

Aromatherapy offers a unique approach to addressing emotional and psychological triggers. Essential oils can influence your mood and mental state, providing a natural means to manage cravings. For instance, the scent of lavender is known for its calming effects, which can alleviate anxiety and reduce the urge to snack mindlessly during stressful moments. By incorporating specific essential oils into your daily routine, you can create an environment that promotes emotional stability and helps mitigate the cravings that often accompany emotional distress.

What is Aromatherapy?

Aromatherapy is a holistic healing practice that harnesses the aromatic properties of essential oils derived from plants. These concentrated extracts are known for their therapeutic benefits, which can enhance physical, emotional, and mental well-being. Aromatherapy offers a natural approach to address these issues. I have found it to be highly effective in combating sugar cravings and addiction. It is also a powerful tool to manage stress and anxiety When essential oils are applied topically, they can penetrate the skin and provide localized benefits, supporting areas of discomfort or tension. Diffusing essential oils in your environment can create a calming atmosphere, setting the stage for relaxation and mindfulness.

Essential oils can be used in numerous ways, including inhalation, topical application, and diffusion. Inhalation allows the scent molecules to travel directly to the brain, influencing the limbic system, which is responsible for emotions and memory.

When it comes to cravings, certain essential oils have been found to help curb unwanted urges and promote a sense of satisfaction. For instance, oils like peppermint and grapefruit are known for their invigorating properties that can help suppress appetite and boost energy. Comforting scents like vanilla and lavender may help reduce stress-induced cravings by promoting relaxation and emotional balance. Understanding the specific properties of different essential oils empowers individuals to select the right blends to support their unique needs and preferences.

Essential Oil Toolkit for Cravings

Sweet Relief Blend

Sweet Relief Blend is a natural and aromatic solution to manage those annoying sugar cravings, especially around your monthly cycle time, while promoting emotional stability and overall health. This unique blend combines essential oils known for their ability to soothe the senses and curb cravings, making it an ideal addition to your aromatherapy toolkit.

The Sweet Relief Blend features a harmonious mix of lavender, geranium, and sweet orange essential oils. Lavender is renowned for its calming properties, helping to ease stress and anxiety that often accompany cravings. By promoting relaxation, lavender can assist in reducing the urge to indulge in unhealthy snacks or comfort foods.

Geranium, on the other hand, is celebrated for its uplifting effects on mood, which can be particularly beneficial for those experiencing emotional eating. Sweet orange adds a delightful, citrusy note that not only brightens the blend but also serves as a natural appetite suppressant, making it a perfect companion in your quest for craving control.

To create your Sweet Relief Blend, start with a base of carrier oil, such as jojoba or sweet almond oil, to dilute the essential oils and make them safe for topical application. Combine 5 drops of lavender, 3 drops of geranium, and 4 drops of sweet orange in a small glass bottle. This recipe can easily be adjusted to suit your personal preferences or sensitivities. Once blended, you can apply it to pulse points like your wrists or temples, or even diffuse it in your living space to fill the air with its soothing aroma.

Incorporating the Sweet Relief Blend into your daily routine can enhance your mindfulness around cravings. Consider using it during moments of temptation or stress, taking a deep breath of the aroma to center yourself. This practice not only helps to curb cravings but also encourages a moment of reflection, allowing you to assess whether the craving stems from physical hunger or emotional triggers. By creating a conscious connection with your cravings, you empower yourself to make healthier choices.

To effectively use essential oils as a tool for managing cravings, it is essential to identify your triggers. Journaling about your cravings can help pinpoint the emotions associated with them. Are you reaching for a snack out of boredom, stress, or sadness? Once you recognize these patterns, you can pair your identified emotions with appropriate essential oils. For example, citrus oils like lemon and orange can energize and uplift your spirit, making them ideal for combating feelings of fatigue or lethargy.

Incorporating aromatherapy into your daily rituals can also provide a proactive approach to craving control. Diffusing essential oils in your home or office can create a positive atmosphere that counters negative emotions. Additionally, using essential oil blends in personal care routines, such as adding a few drops of peppermint oil to your lotion, can provide a refreshing boost that curbs cravings throughout the day. Engaging in mindful practices, such as meditation or yoga, while using these oils can deepen your emotional awareness and further enhance their effectiveness.

Citrus Zest Invigoration

Citrus zest, with its vibrant aroma and invigorating properties, plays a significant role in the realm of aromatherapy. The zest of citrus fruits, such as oranges, lemons, and grapefruits, contain essential oils that are not only uplifting but also have distinct therapeutic benefits. These oils are characterized by their refreshing scent, which can stimulate the senses and promote a sense of alertness, making them an excellent addition to any craving control strategy.

Incorporating citrus zest into your daily routine can provide both psychological and physiological benefits. The bright, fresh fragrance of citrus essential oils can evoke feelings of happiness and positivity, which is crucial if you are navigating the complexities of cravings that often arise from emotional triggers. If you find you regularly experience shifts in mood or energy levels, utilizing citrus zest can serve as a natural mood enhancer, helping to alleviate stress.

One effective technique to maximize the benefits of citrus zest is through the creation of aromatherapy blends. A simple yet powerful recipe involves combining a few drops of lemon essential oil with a carrier oil, such as sweet almond or jojoba oil. This blend can be used for topical application, allowing the invigorating scent to uplift your spirits while also moisturizing the skin. Additionally, diffusing a mixture of citrus oils—like grapefruit, lime, and orange—can fill your space with an energizing aroma, creating an environment that supports mindful eating and craving management.

Beyond mood enhancement, citrus zest is known for its potential to boost metabolism and support digestion. If your goal is weight loss you should also be focusing on maintaining a healthy metabolism. This can be a challenge, but the invigorating properties of citrus oils can provide the necessary support. By integrating citrus zest into your weight loss and maintenance routine, you may find that it helps promote a feeling of fullness and satisfaction, reducing the urge to indulge in unhealthy cravings. This dual action of uplifting the spirit while supporting physical health makes citrus zest a powerful ally in craving control

Chocolate Craving Buster

All of us are subject to chocolate cravings from time to time but is also an addiction for many people. Sugar addiction can lead to a vicious cycle of guilt and regret that will significantly impact weight loss results.

This section, "Chocolate Craving Buster," will explore the intersection of aromatherapy and cravings, and will give you some effective essential oil blends that can help mitigate your desire for chocolate without sacrificing satisfaction.

Research indicates that the sense of smell is intricately linked to our emotions and cravings. Chocolate, with its rich and comforting aroma, often triggers a sense of pleasure and reward in the brain. However, essential oils can provide an alternative sensory experience that may help satisfy your mind's craving for indulgence. Scents like vanilla, bergamot, and sweet orange can evoke similar feelings of comfort and happiness, potentially reducing the desire for chocolate. Incorporating these oils into your daily routine creates a balanced approach to cravings.

To create your own "Chocolate Craving Buster" blend, start with a base of sweet orange essential oil, known for its uplifting properties. Combine it with a few drops of vanilla oil, which adds a creamy, sweet scent reminiscent of chocolate desserts. For an added layer of complexity, consider including a drop of ylang-ylang, which can enhance feelings of relaxation and satisfaction. This blend can be diffused in your living space or applied topically, helping to curb those sudden urges for chocolate.

Using aromatherapy techniques can also be beneficial in managing cravings. When you feel a chocolate craving coming on, take a moment to breathe deeply and inhale your "Chocolate Craving Buster" blend.

Focus on the scent and allow it to envelop you, redirecting your thoughts and desires. Practicing mindfulness in this way not only helps to distract from the craving but also encourages a more conscious decision-making process regarding food choices. I have found this approach to be extremely effective with patients who struggle with sugar addiction.

Balance Blend for Snacking

As we age, our bodies and cravings evolve, making it essential to find ways to maintain a balanced lifestyle. Snacking can become a source of guilt when it leads to unhealthy choices or weight gain. However, with the right approach, snacking can be transformed into a nourishing experience that supports overall well-being.

Aromatherapy harnesses the power of essential oils to influence our mood and well-being. As we navigate the complexities of cravings, certain scents can help us maintain a sense of balance, reducing the desire for unhealthy snacks. Essential oils such as grapefruit and peppermint are known for their appetite-suppressing properties, while oils like lavender and chamomile can soothe emotional eating triggers. By integrating these oils into your snacking routine, you can create a supportive environment that fosters mindful eating habits and reduces impulsive cravings. Creating a "Balance Blend" for snacking involves selecting oils that complement each other to effectively curb cravings while enhancing them. your overall snacking experience. A simple yet effective recipe

includes a combination of grapefruit, peppermint, and sweet orange oils. The citrus notes of grapefruit and sweet orange offer a refreshing aroma that energizes and uplifts, while peppermint provides a cooling sensation that can help suppress appetite. To use this blend, add a few drops to a diffuser while preparing your snacks, or mix with carrier oil to apply to pulse points when the craving strikes.

In addition to using essential oils in the air, incorporating them into your snacks can enhance both flavor and health benefits. For instance, consider drizzling a few drops of lemon or orange essential oil onto fresh fruit or mixed nuts for a zesty flavored boost. Not only do these oils add a delightful taste, but they also provide a sense of satisfaction that can help prevent overindulgence. Furthermore, experimenting with essential oil-infused herbal teas can create a calming ritual that supports mindfulness during your snacking moments.

Satisfying Savory Scent

The desire for comfort and satisfaction can sometimes manifest in cravings for familiar and savory aromas. This subchapter explores how specific essential oils can create a satisfying savory scent that not only delights the senses but also helps to curb cravings, providing a comprehensive approach to maintaining balance in life.

Aromatherapy blends utilizing savory essential oils can evoke feelings of warmth and contentment. Oils such as basil, rosemary, and sage are not only known for their culinary uses but also their aromatic properties that can enhance mood and reduce stress. When inhaled, these scents can trigger memories of home-cooked meals and gatherings, creating a sense of nostalgia that helps mitigate cravings for unhealthy snacks or emotional eating. Incorporating oils into the environment, you can create an atmosphere that promotes relaxation and satisfaction.

To harness the benefits of savory scents, consider creating your essential oil blends. A simple recipe involves combining a few drops of basil essential oil with rosemary and a hint of thyme. This blend can be diffused in your living space or added to a personal inhaler for on-the-go use. The act of inhaling this combination can provide a grounding effect, helping you to feel more centered and less likely to reach for unhealthy food options when cravings strike.

Another effective technique is to incorporate savory essential oils into your cooking. Infusing oils like garlic or oregano into your dishes not only enhances flavor but also fills your kitchen with enticing aromas that can satisfy your senses. The therapeutic properties of these oils can uplift your mood and create a more enjoyable dining experience. This approach encourages mindful eating, allowing you to savor each bite and appreciate the flavors, which can further reduce the likelihood of mindless snacking.

In addition to blending and cooking, using savory scents in self-care rituals can amplify their benefits. Consider adding a few drops of essential oils to your bath or mixing them into body lotions. This practice not only nourishes the skin but also envelops you in a comforting scent that can help alleviate stress and anxiety. By making savory scents a part of your daily routine, you can foster a greater sense of well-being and satisfaction, ultimately supporting your efforts in craving control and achieving a balanced life.

Fiber Booster Aroma

As we age, maintaining a balanced diet becomes increasingly important for overall health and well-being. One of the critical components often overlooked in our daily nutrition is fiber, which plays a significant role in digestion, weight management, and even blood sugar regulation. To support a fiber-rich lifestyle, we can turn to the powerful world of aromatherapy. The "Fiber Booster Aroma" blend is designed not only to uplift your spirits but also to help curb cravings and promote healthy eating habits. This subchapter will explore how specific essential oils can enhance your fiber intake experience, making your journey toward a balanced life more enjoyable and effective.

The Fiber Booster Aroma blend incorporates essential oils known for their appetite-suppressing and digestive-supporting properties. Key ingredients include grapefruit, ginger, and peppermint. Grapefruit essential oil is renowned for its ability to help control cravings and promote feelings of fullness, making it an ideal choice for those looking to manage their weight. Ginger, with its warming properties, aids digestion and can alleviate feelings of bloating or discomfort often associated with dietary changes. Finally, peppermint essential oil is not only refreshing but also has been shown to help reduce hunger pangs and improve overall digestive health, making it a perfect addition to this blend.

Creating your own Fiber Booster Aroma is simple and can become a delightful ritual in your daily routine. Start with a base of carrier oil, such as jojoba or sweet almond oil, which can help dilute the essential oils and make them safe for topical application. Blend 10 drops of grapefruit essential oil, 5 drops of ginger essential oil, and 5 drops of peppermint essential oil into the carrier oil. Mix thoroughly and store the blend in a dark glass bottle to protect it from light degradation. This blend can be used in various ways: as a massage oil on your abdomen to support digestion, in a diffuser to create an uplifting atmosphere, or even as a personal fragrance that encourages mindful eating.

In conjunction with using the Fiber Booster Aroma blend, it's crucial to adopt mindful eating practices. Aromatherapy can enhance awareness of your body's signals, helping you distinguish between true hunger and emotional cravings. Consider using the blend before meals to create a calming environment that encourages you to eat slowly and thoughtfully. Inhaling the aroma of the blend can stimulate your senses, making you more attuned to the flavors and textures of your food, leading to greater satisfaction and reduced overeating.

As you embrace the Fiber Booster Aroma in your daily routine, remember that balance is key. While this blend can support your journey toward healthier eating habits, it should complement a well-rounded diet rich in fiber from whole foods such as fruits, vegetables, whole grains, and legumes. By incorporating this aromatic approach to managing cravings and enhancing digestion, you can cultivate a more balanced life that empowers you to thrive beyond the age of 40. With a little creativity and intention, the Fiber Booster Aroma can become a cherished part of your wellness toolkit.

Calming Lavender Escape

As we navigate the complexities of life, particularly after the age of 40, the need for self-care and stress management becomes increasingly vital. One of the most effective natural remedies for promoting relaxation and reducing cravings is lavender essential oil. Renowned for its calming properties, lavender has been a staple in aromatherapy for centuries, providing a soothing escape from the daily pressures that can lead to unhealthy cravings. This section explores the benefits of lavender and offers practical recipes that harness its power to create a tranquil atmosphere. Lavender essential oil is derived from the Lavandula angustifolia plant, known for its gentle yet effective properties. Research has shown that lavender can help reduce anxiety, improve sleep quality, and enhance overall emotional well-being. For those of you who are over 40, these benefits are particularly important, as life transitions during this period can lead to increased stress and emotional upheaval. By incorporating lavender into your daily routine, you can cultivate a sense of calm that helps mitigate cravings for unhealthy foods or habits often triggered by stress.

To create your calming lavender escape, consider blending lavender essential oil with other complementary oils. A simple yet effective recipe involves mixing three drops of lavender oil with two drops of bergamot and one drop of ylang-ylang. This combination not only enhances the soothing properties of lavender but also adds uplifting notes that can elevate your mood. Use this blend in a diffuser during your evening routine to create a peaceful environment conducive to relaxation and introspection.

Another effective technique to incorporate lavender into your life is through a calming lavender roller blend. Combine ten drops of lavender essential oil with five drops of sweet almond oil in a 10 ml roller bottle. Apply this blend to your wrists, neck, and temples whenever you feel overwhelmed. The act of applying the oil becomes a mindful ritual, allowing you to take a moment for yourself and reset your emotional state. The familiar scent of lavender can serve as a gentle reminder to breathe deeply and let go of stress, reducing the likelihood of indulging in cravings.

In addition to using lavender in blends and rollers, incorporating it into your bath routine can provide a luxurious escape. Add a few drops of lavender essential oil to a warm bath along with Epsom salts for a truly relaxing experience. The heat from the water helps to release the oil's calming properties, allowing you to unwind and reflect. This ritual promotes relaxation but also encourages mindfulness, helping to cultivate a balanced relationship with cravings and emotional well-being. By embracing the calming benefits of lavender, you can create a nurturing environment that supports a healthier, more balanced life carrier oil for a refreshing massage or add a few drops to your bath for a revitalizing soak. The warm water combined with the invigorating

Grounding Earthy Blend

As we navigate the complexities of life, particularly after the age of forty, our bodies and minds often crave balance and stability. The "Grounding Earthy Blend" serves as a powerful tool in achieving this equilibrium using carefully selected essential oils. This unique blend is designed to evoke feelings of security and calmness, making it a perfect companion for those moments when cravings for comfort foods or emotional eating arise. By harnessing the natural properties of grounding oils, individuals can find solace and clarity in their daily routines.

The primary oils in the Grounding Earthy Blend include vetiver, cedarwood, and patchouli. Vetiver, known for its deep calming and grounding qualities, helps to anchor the mind and body, reducing stress and anxiety. Cedarwood, with its warm and woodsy aroma, not only promotes relaxation but also enhances feelings of self-assurance. Patchouli adds an earthy richness to the blend, offering a sense of balance and harmony. Together, these oils create a powerful synergy that can help individuals regain control over their cravings and emotional responses.

To incorporate the Grounding Earthy Blend into your daily life, consider using it in various forms. Diffusing the blend in your living space can create a calming atmosphere, perfect for unwinding after a long day or preparing for a restful night's sleep. Additionally, combining the oils with a carrier oil for topical application can enhance their therapeutic benefits. Applying the blend to pulse points or the soles of your feet can provide immediate grounding effects, especially during moments of stress or temptation. Another effective method for utilizing the Earthy Blend is through meditation and mindfulness practices. Incorporating the blend into your meditation routine can deepen your experience, allowing you.to connect more profoundly with your inner self. As the soothing aromas envelop you, visualize your cravings dissipating, replaced by feelings of calm and centeredness. This practice not only helps in managing immediate urges but also fosters a long-term sense of control over emotional eating.

Probiotics- Another Way to Combat Sugar Cravings

Sugar cravings can be a significant hurdle for those of you experiencing changes in metabolism, hormone levels, and gut health. As we age, our bodies become more susceptible to imbalances within the gut microbiome which can lead to increased cravings for sugar and other unhealthy foods. Understanding the link between gut health and sugar cravings is crucial for anyone who is addicted to sugar. One method I recommend is to use probiotics to help restore the balance of beneficial bacteria in your digestive system.

Probiotics are live microorganisms that, when consumed in adequate amounts, confer health benefits to the host. They play a vital role in maintaining gut health, influencing digestion, and regulating metabolism. Research has shown that the composition of gut bacteria can significantly impact cravings and appetite regulation. By enhancing the diversity and abundance of beneficial bacteria with probiotics, individuals may experience a decrease in sugar cravings, making it easier to resist the temptation to indulge in sugary treats.

One of the key takeaways is that probiotics can help curb sugar cravings by improving gut health and reducing inflammation. An unhealthy gut can lead to dysbiosis, a condition where harmful bacteria outnumber beneficial ones. This imbalance can disrupt the production of neurotransmitters and hormones that regulate mood and appetite, leading to increased cravings for sugary foods. Probiotics can help restore this balance, reducing inflammation in the gut and supporting the production of beneficial compounds that help regulate cravings, leading to healthier eating patterns.

Additionally, probiotics can influence the way our bodies metabolize sugar. Certain strains of probiotics have been shown to enhance insulin sensitivity and improve glucose metabolism. This is particularly important for overweight individuals as insulin resistance tends to increase with age, making it easier to develop sugar cravings and difficult to manage blood sugar levels. By improving insulin sensitivity, probiotics can help stabilize blood sugar levels, reducing the likelihood of sudden cravings for sugary foods and helping individuals maintain consistent energy levels throughout the day.

Incorporating probiotics into your daily routine can be a beneficial strategy for managing sugar cravings and supporting overall health. Options include probiotic-rich foods like yogurt, kefir, sauerkraut, and kimchi, as well as dietary supplements. It is essential to choose high-quality probiotic products that contain effective strains and adequate CFU (colony-forming units) counts to ensure maximum benefits

CHAPTER 9:
Balancing Hormones Naturally

Hormones are a huge topic and one of the leading factors that can impact weight loss. In this subchapter, we will be discussing the hormone imbalances that could slow down your weight loss efforts. Make a list of the hormones that you feel could potentially be a "root cause" of your weight loss struggles.

TIP: If you have not had a full hormone panel or have not had one done in the last 6 months, consider having the tests done asap.

Understanding Hormonal Changes

As you age, your hormonal changes will play a significant role in your weight loss journey. Hormones such as estrogen, progesterone, and testosterone fluctuate during various stages of life, affecting metabolism, energy level, and the way the body stores and burns fat. It is important to understand these hormonal changes to effectively manage your weight.

One of the key hormonal changes that we can experience is a decrease in estrogen levels. This decline in estrogen can lead to weight gain, particularly around the abdomen. Estrogen helps regulate metabolism and energy levels. When levels decrease, you may notice a decrease in your energy levels and an increase in fat storage. Understanding how estrogen impacts weight gain can help you make informed choices and take control of your body. In addition to estrogen, progesterone levels also fluctuate during various stages of life. Progesterone is essential for maintaining a healthy metabolism and can affect how the body processes carbohydrates and fats. Progesterone levels tend to decrease as we age, which can lead to weight gain and difficulty losing weight.

Having a good understanding of the role of progesterone in weight management, you can make the necessary adjustments to your diet and exercise routine to support overall hormonal balance.

Testosterone is another hormone that plays a role in weight loss. While testosterone is often associated with men, women also produce lesser amounts of this hormone. Testosterone helps build muscle mass and increase metabolism, making it easier to burn fat and maintain a healthy weight. As women age, testosterone levels naturally decline, which can make it more challenging to build and maintain muscle mass. By understanding the role of testosterone in weight management, women can incorporate strength training exercises into their routines to support their hormonal balance.

Insulin is a hormone that regulates blood sugar levels and helps the body store and use glucose for energy. When insulin levels are high, the body is more likely to store fat, especially around the abdomen. This can make it harder to lose weight, as insulin resistance becomes more common with age. Watch the sugars, track your food intake, and check the ingredients for sources of sugar that could be spiking your insulin and slowing down your weight loss.

TIP: The easiest way to balance insulin is through the food that you are ingesting. Eat with a focus on stabilizing blood sugar levels.

Cortisol- is another hormone that can impact weight loss. Also known as stress hormones. Elevated levels of cortisol can lead to increased appetite cravings for unhealthy foods, and weight gain, particularly around the midsection. Managing stress levels through relaxation techniques, exercise, and adequate sleep can help balance your cortisol levels and support your weight loss goals. One of the primary roles of cortisol is to help the body respond to stress. When faced with a stressful situation, cortisol levels rise, providing a burst of energy by increasing glucose availability and enhancing the body's ability to use carbohydrates, fats, and proteins. However, chronic stress can lead to prolonged elevated levels of cortisol, which may disrupt normal bodily functions. For women over fifty, this is particularly relevant as hormonal fluctuations during menopause can exacerbate stress responses, making it more challenging to maintain a healthy weight and metabolic balance.

Elevated cortisol levels are intricately linked to weight gain, especially in the abdominal area. "Stress belly. "This phenomenon occurs because cortisol promotes fat storage and can increase cravings for high-calorie foods, particularly those rich in sugar and fat. Hormonal changes can lead to a natural increase in body fat while also decreasing muscle mass, further complicating weight loss efforts. Understanding the relationship between cortisol and body composition is essential for people navigating hormonal shifts and seeking to improve their health.

Prolonged elevated levels of cortisol can lead to other health issues beyond weight gain, including increased risk of heart disease, osteoporosis, and cognitive decline. Stress management becomes crucial in mitigating these risks. Incorporating practices such as mindfulness, regular physical activity, and adequate sleep can help regulate cortisol levels. Leptin is a hormone primarily produced by adipose (fat) tissue that plays a crucial role in regulating energy balance by inhibiting hunger, thereby helping to maintain body weight. In a healthy metabolic state, leptin communicates with the brain to signal when we have enough energy stored and when it is time to eat. However, many women experience a phenomenon known as leptin resistance and do not realize it. This is where the brain becomes less responsive to the signals sent by leptin. This condition can lead to persistent feelings of hunger, reduced energy expenditure, and weight gain, creating a cycle that can be difficult to break.

The relationship between leptin resistance and weight gain is multifaceted and, in my experience, it has shown to be a common problem but is often overlooked by conventional medicine. When leptin levels are chronically elevated due to excess body fat, the brain may begin to ignore the hormone's signals. This insensitivity can result from several factors, including inflammation, hormonal imbalances, and lifestyle choices such as poor diet and lack of physical activity. As leptin resistance develops, the body's ability to regulate appetite and energy use diminishes, leading to increased caloric intake and decreased metabolic efficiency. For women, who often face unique hormonal fluctuations throughout their lives, the impact of leptin resistance can be particularly pronounced.

Leptin Resistance and Inflammation in the Body

One of the contributing factors to leptin resistance is the presence of inflammation in the body. Chronic inflammation can stem from a diet high in processed foods, sugar, and unhealthy fats, which can interfere with leptin signaling. This is particularly concerning for women, who may be more susceptible to inflammatory conditions due to hormonal changes related to menstruation, pregnancy, and menopause. For men with diabetes or cardiovascular disease, understanding the inflammatory pathways involved in leptin resistance is essential to not only help you decrease inflammation for weight loss but also to regain control over your metabolic health and combat unwanted belly fat.

Ghrelin

Think of can think of ghrelin as your hunger hormone. Like the other hunger hormone, Leptin, it communicates with the brain- in this case, telling your brain to eat. Every time your stomach becomes empty, it naturally releases ghrelin into your bloodstream. Ghrelin levels are lowered, just after you have finished a meal. They are at their highest when the stomach is empty, and you are ready for your next meal. This scenario is normal when a person is on a healthy diet and maintaining an optimal, healthy weight. An overweight person, on the other hand, will find that -like other hormones, we have explored- ghrelin levels are typically out of order. In most healthy-weight individuals, ghrelin levels decrease in a way that states them and signals their brains to stop eating. However, in obese individuals, ghrelin levels do not decrease enough after eating, which fails to send the brain the signal it needs to stop eating and feel satisfied.

How To Balance Ghrelin Levels

If you have a suspicion your ghrelin levels need a little TLC:

Eat an adequate amount of protein. Protein helps you feel full and should be consumed with every meal.

Avoid sugar as much as possible. As you know by now, consuming too much sugar disrupts hormone balance, making weight loss seem an impossible feat.

How Herbs Can Balance Hormones

One of the primary advantages of herbal remedies is their holistic nature. Unlike conventional medications, which often focus on alleviating symptoms, herbal medicine aims to restore balance within the body. This integrated approach recognizes that hormonal imbalances can be influenced by various factors, including diet, lifestyle, and emotional health. By incorporating herbal remedies into a comprehensive wellness plan and target weight loss approach I have found that we will not only address specific hormonal issues that are affecting the body but also the underlying factors contributing to our overall health. Hormonal balance is a critical aspect of health, particularly for women over forty, as they navigate the transitional phases of menopause and perimenopause. As hormone levels fluctuate, many experience a range of symptoms, including weight gain, mood swings, and fatigue. While conventional treatments often focus on synthetic hormone replacement therapies, an increasing number of women are turning towards herbal remedies as a natural alternative for regulating hormones. Understanding how specific herbs can influence hormonal balance is essential for those seeking to manage these changes effectively and holistically.

One of the most well-known herbs that I recommend my patients use for supporting hormonal health is black cohosh. Traditionally used by Native Americans, this herb is well known for its ability to alleviate menopausal symptoms, including hot flashes and night sweats. Black cohosh works by interacting with estrogen receptors in the body, potentially helping to balance estrogen levels. This makes it particularly beneficial for women experiencing estrogen dominance or imbalance. Incorporating black cohosh into a daily regimen may provide relief from uncomfortable symptoms while promoting overall hormonal equilibrium.

Another powerful herb is chaste tree berry, also known as Vitex. This herb has been used for centuries to address various hormonal issues, particularly those related to the menstrual cycle and premenstrual syndrome (PMS). Chaste tree berry works by stimulating the pituitary gland to produce luteinizing hormone (LH), which can help regulate.

TIP: Chasteberry is my favorite herb to recommend for relieving intense or debilitating cramps during cycle time. Most of my patients have found this to be as helpful as ibuprofen.

Adaptogenic herbs like ashwagandha and rhodiola are also gaining recognition for their ability to support hormonal balance. These herbs help the body adapt to stress, which can significantly impact hormonal health. Chronic stress leads to elevated cortisol levels, disrupting the delicate balance of sex hormones. By managing stress responses, ashwagandha and rhodiola can help maintain hormonal stability, thus supporting weight management and overall health.

Key Herbs for Hormonal Regulation & Managing Menopause

Black Cohosh: Alleviating Menopausal Symptoms

Black cohosh, a perennial herb native to North America, has gained recognition as a natural remedy for alleviating menopausal symptoms. Navigating the hormonal fluctuations of midlife can be challenging, often accompanied by symptoms such as hot flashes, night sweats, mood swings, and sleep disturbances. As many seek alternatives to hormone replacement therapy, black cohosh presents a compelling option, particularly for those interested in herbal remedies and natural supplements.

Red Clover: Phytoestrogen and Heart Health

Red clover plays a unique role in balancing hormones, especially for women over 40 who may be experiencing the challenges of hormonal fluctuations associated with perimenopause and menopause. Understanding how red clover works can empower women to take control of their health as they navigate this transitional phase of life.

Phytoestrogens are plant-derived compounds that mimic estrogen in the body, offering a natural alternative for those seeking hormone balance without the use of synthetic hormones. Red clover contains several types of isoflavones, including genistein and daidzein, which have been studied for their ability to bind to estrogen receptors. For women experiencing symptoms such as hot flashes, night sweats, and mood swings, incorporating red clover into their health regimen may provide relief by moderating estrogen levels and alleviating these discomforts. This can be particularly beneficial for women who are looking for natural solutions to hormonal imbalances.

In addition to its role in hormone regulation, red clover has been linked to cardiovascular health. As women age, the risk of heart disease increases, often exacerbated by hormonal changes. Research suggests that the isoflavones found in red clover may help improve arterial function and lower cholesterol levels, thereby contributing to better heart health. By promoting healthy blood flow and reducing LDL cholesterol, red clover can be an integral part of a holistic approach to maintaining cardiovascular wellness during midlife.

Vitex (Chaste Tree): Balancing Progesterone Levels

Vitex, commonly known as chaste tree, has long been revered in herbal medicine for its ability to support hormonal balance, particularly in women over 40 navigating the complexities of midlife. As hormonal fluctuations become more pronounced during this stage, many women experience symptoms linked to progesterone deficiency, such as irregular menstrual cycles, mood swings, and weight gain. Vitex serves as a natural remedy, promoting the body's production of progesterone while helping to alleviate these distressing symptoms.

One of the primary mechanisms through which Vitex operates is its influence on the pituitary gland, which plays a crucial role in hormone regulation. By stimulating the pituitary gland, Vitex enhances the secretion of luteinizing hormone (LH), which in turn promotes ovulation and the production of progesterone from the ovaries. This is particularly beneficial for women experiencing anovulation or irregular cycles due to age-related hormonal shifts. As the body begins to balance its progesterone levels, many women report improvements in mood stability, reduced premenstrual symptoms, and a more predictable menstrual cycle.

In addition to its hormonal balancing effects, Vitex has been shown to address various symptoms associated with hormonal imbalances. For instance, many struggle with weight management as metabolic rates slow and hormonal levels fluctuate. By restoring progesterone levels, Vitex may help mitigate weight gain that can occur due to hormonal shifts, particularly around menopause. Furthermore, its adaptogenic properties can help reduce stress, another factor that often exacerbates hormonal imbalances and weight issues in this demographic.

Dong Quai: The Female Ginseng

Dong Quai, often referred to as the "female ginseng," has gained recognition in the realm of herbal remedies, particularly for its potential benefits in regulating hormones and addressing hormonal imbalances in women over 40. This powerful herb, native to China, has been utilized for centuries in traditional Chinese medicine to promote women's health. Its adaptogenic properties help the body respond to stress and maintain balance, making it an appealing option for those navigating the often-tumultuous changes that accompany midlife.

In addition to its hormonal benefits, Dong Quai may also play a role in weight management, an important aspect for many women over 40. As hormonal changes can lead to weight gain, particularly around the abdomen, incorporating Dong Quai into a comprehensive approach to health can be beneficial. The herb supports healthy blood circulation and may enhance metabolic processes, which can contribute to more effective weight loss efforts. When combined with a balanced diet and regular exercise, Dong Quai can be a valuable addition to a weight loss regimen.

Maca Root: Enhancing Libido and Energy

Maca root, a powerful adaptogen native to the Andes mountains of Peru, has gained significant attention in recent years for its potential benefits in enhancing libido and energy, particularly among women over forty. This age group often experiences hormonal fluctuations that can lead to decreased sexual desire and fatigue, among other symptoms. Maca root, scientifically known as Lepidium meyenii, is rich in essential nutrients and bioactive compounds that may help balance hormones, thereby supporting overall vitality and sexual health.

For women who are overweight, experiencing a low libido can impact relationships due to how it makes us feel about ourselves. Excess weight makes us feel self-conscious during intimate moments with a partner, further intensifying the focus on weight issues. This is a common concern for many of my patients and most have reported back that intimacy does return as they lose weight and supplement Maca. Maca influences the endocrine system, promoting balanced hormone production that can lead to improved libido and sexual function. Maca also plays a role in alleviating symptoms of menopause, such as hot flashes and mood swings, which can further impact sexual desire. By supporting hormonal balance, maca may help women navigate this transitional phase more comfortably. Moreover, it has been suggested that maca can increase levels of certain hormones, such as estrogen and testosterone, which are crucial for maintaining sexual health. This ability to support hormonal equilibrium makes maca an appealing option for women seeking natural remedies for libido enhancement and energy support.

One of the key components of maca root is its rich profile of amino acids, vitamins, and minerals. These nutrients work synergistically to improve energy levels and enhance mood, which can be particularly beneficial for women facing the challenges of midlife hormonal changes. Regular consumption of maca has been linked to increased stamina and endurance, making it a popular choice for those looking to combat fatigue often associated with hormonal imbalances. When we feel energetic and strong on the inside, it also becomes easier to stay on track with weight loss goals.

Testimonials from my Patients on Balancing Hormones with Herbs

I always like to share my testimonials from some of my women patients who have successfully navigated the complexities of hormonal imbalances and often provide invaluable insights into the efficacy of herbal remedies and lifestyle changes. They serve as both inspiration and evidence that natural solutions can be effective in addressing these issues.

One compelling testimonial is from a client Linda, a 52-year-old who struggled with unexplained weight gain for years. After trying various diets and medications without lasting success, she turned to herbal remedies. Linda incorporated supplements such as black cohosh and chaste tree berries into her daily routine, alongside a balanced diet rich in whole foods and proteins. Within a few months, she noticed not only a reduction in her weight but also improvements in her energy levels and

Another profound account comes from Sarah, who experienced severe symptoms of perimenopause, including weight gain around her abdomen and fatigue. Frustrated with conventional treatments, I recommended that she begin using a blend of quai and maca root while also practicing mindfulness and yoga. She found that these herbs not only helped her manage her weight but also alleviated some of the emotional turmoil associated with hormonal fluctuations. This in turn helped her lessen the frequency of her emotional eating habits. Her experience underscores the importance of a multifaceted approach when dealing with hormonal imbalances, combining both physical, nutritional, and mental health strategies.

In a unique experience, Maria, a 46-year-old, shares how herbal teas became a staple in her journey toward hormonal health. I recommended a mix of herbal teas, and she began drinking a daily infusion of nettle and raspberry leaf. Over time, Maria observed a gradual decrease in bloating and cravings, which significantly aided her weight loss efforts. This testimonial highlights the potential of simple nutrition adjustments she made, such as incorporating herbal teas, to impact hormonal health positively. Maria's story serves as a reminder that small, consistent changes can lead to significant improvements in well-being and weight loss. I hope the collective examples of my patients reveal a common theme: the power of herbal remedies in addressing the multifaceted challenges of hormonal imbalances.

While individual results may vary, I hope the testimonials provide hope and motivation for those of you facing similar struggles. By sharing their journeys, these women not only validate the effectiveness of natural solutions but also empower others to explore herbal remedies as a viable path toward achieving hormonal balance and weight loss in midlife. As more women seek alternatives to conventional treatments, these stories. serve as a guiding light, illustrating that balance is achievable through natural means.

Menopause

One of the most noticeable physical changes during menopause is weight gain, particularly around the abdomen. This redistribution of body fat is attributed to hormonal fluctuations. As estrogen levels decline, the body begins to store fat in the abdominal area rather than the hips and thighs, leading to an increased risk of visceral fat accumulation. This type of fat is associated with various health risks, including heart disease and type 2 diabetes. Women may find that despite maintaining their usual diet and exercise routines, weight loss becomes more challenging, underscoring the importance of adjusting lifestyle habits to counteract these changes.

In addition to weight gain, menopause can trigger a variety of other physical symptoms that can indirectly influence weight loss efforts. Hot flashes, night sweats, and sleep disturbances are common complaints that can disrupt daily routines and affect energy levels. Poor sleep can lead to increased cravings for high-calorie foods and decreased motivation for physical activity. Mood swings and anxiety, which can accompany hormonal changes, may lead many women to seek comfort in food, making it even harder to achieve or maintain a hey weight.

Mood Instability

One of the most common emotional responses that I see to hormonal changes is mood instability. Many clients report feelings of irritability, sadness, or frustration, which can be exacerbated by the physical symptoms associated with hormonal fluctuations, such as hot flashes and sleep disturbances. These mood shifts can create a cycle where emotional distress leads to unhealthy coping mechanisms, such as overeating or neglecting physical activity. Emotional eating and menopause symptoms are connected. Recognizing this link between emotional health and hormonal balance is vital for people who struggle with weight loss because addressing emotional eating habits can enhance their overall health outcomes.

Anxiety is another prevalent issue that I see with patients who are experiencing hormonal imbalances. The decline in estrogen can contribute to increased levels of anxiety, making everyday stressors feel overwhelming. This heightened state of anxiety not only affects mental health but can also impact physical health behaviors. Some may find themselves feeling too anxious to engage in regular exercise or to prepare healthy meals, opting instead for convenience foods that are often high in calories and soothing the negative emotional state or symptoms they are experiencing. To counter these effects, it is crucial to implement strategies that promote emotional stability, such as mindfulness practices, therapy, or support groups.

Depression is a serious concern linked to hormonal changes during this life stage. Many women experience depressive symptoms as their bodies go through significant shifts. The relationship between hormones and mood is complex, and the interplay between declining hormone levels and life changes—such as retirement, loss of loved ones, or shifts in family dynamics—can exacerbate feelings of sadness or hopelessness and is a leading contributor to weight gain. Women need to seek help when experiencing these symptoms, as untreated depression can lead to more health complications. Engaging with healthcare providers to explore treatment options can empower women to take control of their emotional health.

Thyroid Dysfunction

Thyroid health is a common root cause of weight issues because hormonal changes during menopause can exacerbate the effects of an underactive or overactive thyroid. The thyroid gland, located at the base of the neck, plays a crucial role in regulating metabolism, energy levels, and overall hormonal balance. When the thyroid does not produce sufficient hormones (hypothyroidism) or produces too much (hyperthyroidism), it can lead to a variety of health issues, including weight gain, fatigue, and mood disturbances, all of which can be particularly challenging during the menopausal transition.

Thyroid health plays a crucial role in regulating metabolism, making it an essential topic for women, especially those grappling with leptin resistance. The thyroid gland, located in the neck, produces hormones that control various bodily functions, including how the body uses energy. When the thyroid is functioning optimally, it helps maintain a healthy metabolic rate, allowing women to manage their weight effectively and support overall wellness. However, conditions such as hypothyroidism can lead to a slowed metabolism, exacerbating issues related to leptin resistance and making weight management more challenging. Research indicates that women are more prone to thyroid disorders than men, particularly autoimmune conditions like Hashimoto's thyroiditis.

These conditions can lead to lower levels of thyroid hormones, contributing to symptoms such as fatigue, weight gain, and depression. In the context of leptin resistance, thyroid dysfunction can intensify cravings and hunger signals due to the disrupted communication between the thyroid and the leptin feedback loop. Understanding this connection is vital for women aiming to conquer leptin resistance and achieve lifelong weight management.

Nutrition and thyroid health go hand in hand. Approach your diet with a "food as medicine" approach because certain nutrients that your body needs to make thyroid hormones will help increase or decrease thyroid function. Before you start taking drugs, check to see if your diet is missing a crucial piece of your thyroid puzzle, or if you are overindulging in foods that could aggravate it.

TIP: When your thyroid functions at optimum levels with natural methods, you can avoid medication, and weight loss is much easier.

Boost Your Thyroid Function Before Making the Decision to Start Medication

Consider integrating the following herbs, foods, and supplements into your routine if you have hypothyroid issues that are affecting your weight loss attempts.

Iodine -Iodine is an essential mineral for the creation of thyroid hormones and our key dietary sources include iodized salt, seaweed, seafood, and some multivitamins. Are you getting any iodine? Have you recently switched multivitamins or brands of salt and inadvertently eliminated them from your diet? Lack of iodine instigates thyroid disease and weight issues.

Kelp- Seaweed is a potent source of not just iodine but also other minerals, including calcium, iron, and selenium. Seaweed can profoundly increase thyroid function. Add a little bit to soups, broths, and other dishes.

Selenium – helps your thyroid more effectively manufacture hormones and facilitates the transformation of inactive T4 into T3. Just one or two Brazil nuts a day can provide enough selenium.

Ashwagandha -Ashwagandha simultaneously calms and energizes, has benefits for autoimmune disease and inflammation, and increases T3 and T4 production.

Bacopa, and guggul. Bacopa boosts T4 production, but not active T3. It also enhances brain function, enhances memory, and quells anxiety. Guggul improves the conversion of T4 to active T3 and is used for weight loss and high cholesterol.

Tyrosine- An amino acid that serves as a building block for thyroid hormones. You should be able to get it from your diet (poultry, fish, cheese, nuts, and seeds), and your body can make it from other amino acids so be sure to eat enough protein.

Medium-chain triglycerides (MCTs) Coconut oil supports thyroid function by decreasing inflammation, boosting metabolism, and improving thyroid hormone function.

Foods and Herbs That Inhibit Thyroid Function

If you have hyperthyroid disease avoid eating excessive amounts of the following foods and herbs. People with hyperthyroid disease often feel strung out, so it is handy that herbs downregulate thyroid hormones and bring the nervous system down a notch.

Lemon balm, motherwort, and bugleweed- Whether as a single herb or a trio blend, these herbs inhibit hyperthyroid function through a variety of mechanisms, including binding TSH receptors, inhibiting thyroid hormone production, and preventing thyroid hormone conversion from T4 to T3. Lemon balm also prevents autoantibodies from binding to TSH receptors.

Estrogen and Weight Loss

Estrogen deficiency is a common issue that many women face as they approach and transition through menopause. Estrogen, a crucial hormone in the female body, plays a significant role in regulating various physiological processes. As estrogen levels decline, women often experience a range of symptoms, including hot flashes, mood swings, and changes in libido. These fluctuations not only affect overall well-being but can also significantly impact weight management. Understanding the intricacies of estrogen deficiency is essential for women seeking to navigate this phase of life while losing/maintaining a healthy weight.

Low Libido – This is a common issue for men and women who are overweight. Recommended herbal supplements:

Men Formula- Gaia Herbs Male Libido

Women Formula – Designs for Health Libido Stim F

The relationship between estrogen and weight is complex. Estrogen helps to regulate metabolism and fat distribution in the body. During periods of estrogen deficiency, women may notice an increase in abdominal fat, a shift in body composition, and a decrease in muscle mass. This can lead to a frustrating cycle where weight gain becomes more pronounced, further exacerbating feelings of discomfort and dissatisfaction. Recognizing how estrogen influences fat storage and metabolism can empower women to take the initiative in managing their weight during this transitional phase.

In addition to affecting body fat distribution, estrogen deficiency can also impact appetite regulation. Research suggests that estrogen interacts with the brain's hunger centers, influencing how much food we consume and how we feel about it. With lower estrogen levels, women may experience increased cravings, particularly for high-calorie, sugary foods. This change in appetite can make it more challenging to adhere to a healthy diet, contributing to unwanted weight gain. Therefore, understanding the hormonal influences on appetite can help women make more mindful eating choices.

Progesterone levels also decline during this period, which can contribute to mood swings and increased stress levels. The connection between stress and weight gain is well-documented, as stress hormones like cortisol can lead to cravings for unhealthy foods and encourage fat storage, especially in the abdominal area. Furthermore, fluctuations in progesterone can disrupt sleep patterns, leading to fatigue and decreased motivation to engage in physical activity. This cycle of hormonal imbalance, stress, and weight gain underscores the importance of addressing mental and emotional health alongside physical changes.

Nutrient Balancing for Balanced Hormones

Omega-3 fatty acids are crucial for maintaining hormonal balance. Found in fatty fish: salmon, walnuts, and flaxseeds, omega-3s help reduce inflammation and support brain health, which is closely tied to hormonal regulation. These healthy fats play a role in producing hormones like estrogen and progesterone, which can decrease during menopause. Including omega-3-rich foods in your diet can help alleviate symptoms associated with hormonal imbalances, such as mood swings and weight fluctuations. Do not be afraid of eating healthy fat – it will not make you far if you are practicing good portion control. A visual for a healthy fat serving for a woman is your thumb- for a man- serving size is 2 thumbs (2 Tablespoons)

Eating a variety of nutrient-dense foods can help regulate hormone levels and support overall health. Include plenty of fruits, vegetables, lean proteins, and healthy fats in your meals. Avoid processed foods, sugary snacks, and excessive caffeine, disrupting hormone balance, and hindering weight loss efforts.

Muscle mass is a key component of metabolism, as muscle tissue burns more calories at rest compared to fat tissue. After age 50, we can experience a gradual decline in muscle mass, a condition known as sarcopenia. This loss of muscle can be exacerbated by hormonal imbalances, particularly decreased levels of sex hormones. As muscle mass diminishes, the metabolic rate decreases, leading to potential weight gain and increased difficulty in losing unwanted fat. Recognizing the importance of preserving muscle through appropriate lifestyle choices can help mitigate these effects.

Stress management is also crucial for hormone balance. Chronic stress can disrupt hormone levels, leading to weight gain, fatigue, and other health issues. Practice relaxation techniques such as deep breathing, meditation, yoga, or tai chi to help reduce stress and promote hormone balance. Make the time to be available for self-care activities that you enjoy, such as reading, listening to music, or spending time in nature.

Adequate sleep_Getting an adequate amount of sleep is essential for hormone balance and weight loss. Lack of sleep can disrupt hormone levels, leading to increased hunger, cravings, and weight gain. Aim for 7-9 hours of **quality** sleep per night to support hormone balance and overall health. Create a relaxing bedtime routine, such as taking a warm bath, reading a book, or practicing mindfulness, to help you fall asleep easily and improve the quality of your sleep.

PCOS

Scientists have recently discovered a remarkable connection between insulin and reproductive health. The more glucose spikes in our diet, the higher our insulin levels and the higher the incidence of infertility.

When it comes to female infertility, polycystic ovarian syndrome (PCOS) is often to blame. One in eight women experience it and when they do, their ovaries become burdened with cysts and no longer ovulate. PCOS is a disease caused by too much insulin. The more insulin is present, the more PCOS symptoms. Many women with PCOS also have a hard time losing weight because where there is too much insulin, there is an inability to burn fat.

In conclusion, achieving hormone balance is crucial for supporting weight loss goals and overall health. By focusing on a balanced diet, regular exercise, stress management, and adequate sleep, you can help regulate hormone levels and support your weight loss efforts. Incorporate these tips into your daily routine to achieve optimal hormonal balance and feel slim and strong at any age

CHAPTER 10:
Sleep and Stress Management

Importance of Quality Sleep

Quality sleep plays a significant role in weight management for women. When we are sleep-deprived, our bodies produce more ghrelin, the hunger hormone, and less leptin, the hormone that signals fullness. This imbalance can lead to increased cravings and overeating, making it more difficult to stick to a healthy eating plan.

In the quest for weight loss, one often overlooked factor is the importance of quality sleep. Life is busy for everyone these days, and some days we may find ourselves juggling multiple responsibilities, which can lead to disruption or inadequate sleep. However, prioritizing sleep is crucial for our overall health and weight loss goals. Lack of quality sleep can also impact on our metabolism. When we are sleep-deprived, our bodies are less able to efficiently process and burn calories. This can result in weight gain or make it harder to lose weight, even when we are following a balanced diet and exercise routine.In addition, quality sleep is essential for our mental and emotional well-being. When we are well-rested, we are better equipped to manage stress and make healthier choices throughout the day. On the other hand, sleep deprivation can lead to increased levels of cortisol, the stress hormone, which can contribute to weight gain and hinder our weight loss efforts.

Meal Timing Affects Sleep Quality

Meal timing plays a significant role in weight management, and slows with age, understanding how when we eat can influence our body's ability to manage weight becomes increasingly important. Research suggests that aligning mealtimes with the body's natural circadian rhythms can enhance metabolic processes and support weight loss efforts. This subchapter explores the critical connection between meal timing, stress reduction, and effective weight management.

One of the primary factors affecting weight management is insulin sensitivity, which tends to decline with age. Eating at irregular intervals can lead to spikes in insulin levels, promoting fat storage rather than fat burning. By establishing a consistent eating schedule, individuals can help regulate their insulin levels, thereby improving their body's ability to utilize stored fat for energy. This approach not only aids in weight management but can also contribute to more stable energy levels throughout the day, which is crucial for maintaining an active lifestyle—a key component of stress reduction.

Furthermore, the timing of meals can have implications for sleep quality, which is essential for effective weight management. Consuming heavy meals late in the evening can disrupt sleep patterns and lead to poor-quality rest. This can create a vicious cycle, as inadequate sleep often results in increased cravings for high-calorie foods and a decrease in motivation to engage in physical activity. By adopting earlier mealtimes and focusing on lighter, nutrient-dense foods in the evening, individuals can improve their sleep quality, thereby enhancing their overall well-being and supporting their weight loss goals.

Additionally, intermittent fasting has gained popularity as a strategy for weight management among those over 40. This approach involves cycling between periods of eating and fasting, which can help the body become more efficient at burning fat. Research indicates that intermittent fasting can improve metabolic health, reduce inflammation, and even promote cellular repair processes. By incorporating this eating pattern into their lifestyle, individuals can create a structured routine that not only aids in weight management but also aligns with stress reduction principles, providing a sense of control and discipline.

Managing Stress for Weight Loss

In the journey to weight loss, managing stress levels is a crucial component that is often overlooked but can have a significant impact on your overall health and well-being. Stress can lead to emotional eating, lack of motivation to exercise, and hormone imbalances that can hinder weight loss efforts. Therefore, it is important to implement strategies to effectively manage stress to achieve your weight loss goals.

One effective way to manage stress levels is through regular exercise. Exercise has been shown to reduce stress and anxiety levels by releasing feel-good hormones called endorphins. Additionally, physical activity can help improve your mood, increase energy levels, and boost self-confidence, all of which are key factors in maintaining a healthy weight. Aim to incorporate at least 30 minutes of moderate-intensity exercise into your daily routine to help combat stress and improve your overall well-being.

Another important aspect of managing stress levels is practicing relaxation techniques such as deep breathing, meditation, or yoga. These practices can help calm the mind, reduce muscle tension, and promote a sense of inner peace. By taking time to relax and unwind, you can better cope with the daily stressors of life and prevent emotional eating or other unhealthy coping mechanisms that can sabotage your weight loss efforts.

In addition to exercise and relaxation techniques, it is important to prioritize self-care and make time for activities that bring you joy and relaxation. Whether it is reading a book, taking a bubble bath, or spending time with loved ones, finding ways to unwind and recharge can help reduce stress levels and improve your mental and emotional well-being. Remember that self-care is not selfish but essential for maintaining a healthy lifestyle and achieving your weight loss goals.

Managing stress levels is a key component of successful weight loss. By incorporating regular exercise, relaxation techniques, and self-care practices into your daily routine, you can effectively reduce stress, improve your overall well-being, and increase your chances of achieving your weight loss goals. Remember to prioritize your mental and emotional health as you work towards a healthier, happier you.

Relaxation Techniques

In today's fast-paced world, stress is a common factor that can hinder weight loss efforts. It is important to incorporate relaxation techniques into your daily routine to help manage stress levels and promote overall well-being. By taking time to relax and unwind, you will not only improve your mental health but also support your weight loss journey.

One effective relaxation technique is deep breathing exercises. By focusing on your breath and taking slow, deep inhales and exhales, you can calm your mind and body. Deep breathing can help reduce cortisol levels, which is a hormone that can promote weight gain, especially around the abdomen. Incorporating deep breathing exercises into your daily routine can help you relax and de-stress, which can support your weight loss goals.

Another relaxation technique to consider is meditation. Meditation has been shown to reduce stress, improve focus, and promote overall well-being. By taking just a few minutes a day to meditate, you can clear your mind and create a sense of calm. This can help you make better choices when it comes to food and exercise, supporting your weight loss efforts.

There are many guided meditation apps and videos available that can help you get started with meditation practice. Many women find it difficult to try meditation because it requires them to slow down and focus on themselves. Women typically have trouble because we typically, do not put us on our priority list.

Yoga is another great relaxation technique that can benefit women who are looking to lose weight. Yoga combines physical movement with mindfulness and breath work, creating a holistic approach to relaxation. Practicing yoga regularly can help improve flexibility, reduce stress, and promote a sense of well-being. There are many distinctive styles of yoga to choose from, so you can find a practice that suits your preferences and fitness level.

In addition to deep breathing, meditation, and yoga, many other relaxation techniques can support weight loss. Some other options to consider include progressive muscle relaxation, aromatherapy, and spending time in nature. Finding a relaxation technique that works for

you and incorporating it into your daily routine can help you manage stress, improve your mood, and support your weight loss goals. Remember, taking care of your mental and emotional well-being is just as important as taking care of your physical health.

CHAPTER 11:
Supplements and Support

Essential Supplements for Women Over 50

As women age, their bodies undergo various changes that can make it harder to maintain a healthy weight. One way to support your weight loss journey and overall health is by incorporating essential supplements into your daily routine. In this subchapter, we will discuss some of the key supplements that you should consider adding to your diet to support your weight loss goals and overall well-being.

One essential supplement is calcium. As we age, we are at a higher risk for osteoporosis, a condition that weakens bones and increases the risk of fractures. Calcium is important for maintaining strong bones and reducing the risk of osteoporosis. In addition to supporting bone health, calcium has also been shown to aid in weight loss by promoting fat metabolism and reducing fat absorption in the body. The best form of calcium to take is calcium citrate for optimum absorption.

Another important supplement is vitamin D3. Vitamin D3 is crucial for bone health, immune function, and overall well-being. As we age, our bodies become less efficient at producing vitamin D3 from sunlight, making it important to supplement with this essential nutrient. Studies have shown that vitamin D3 deficiency is linked to weight gain and obesity, so ensuring you are getting an adequate amount of this vitamin D3 is crucial for supporting your weight loss goals.

Omega-3 fatty acids are another essential supplement, especially for those of us over fifty. These healthy fats are known for their anti-inflammatory properties and have been shown to support heart health, brain function, and weight loss. Omega-3 fatty acids can help reduce inflammation in the body, joint pain, and bloating. Incorporating omega-3 fatty acids into your diet through supplements or foods like fatty fish, flaxseeds, and walnuts can help support your overall health and weight loss goals.

Probiotics are also important supplements. These beneficial bacteria help support gut health, digestion, and immune function. As we age, our gut health can become compromised, leading to digestive issues and weight gain. Probiotics can help restore the balance of beneficial bacteria in the gut, which can aid in digestion and support weight loss including probiotic-rich foods like yogurt, kefir, and sauerkraut in your diet, or taking high-quality probiotics can help support your weight loss journey and overall health for women.

B-COMPLEX- For weight loss, be sure to get a superior quality full B-B-Complex and not just B12. All the B vitamins are important for fat metabolism, and energy production.

Another thing to consider is the quality of supplements you are putting into your body. Avoid buying supplements that are cheaper because they are cheaper for a reason. Just as we need to be label detectives with our food shipping, unfortunately, manufacturers of herbal supplements also put added sugars and chemicals into their products as well.

TIP: Do not take too many supplements. Supplements are meant to "supplement" our diet, not be the main meal.

Seeking Professional Help

Seeking professional help on your weight loss journey can be a game-changer for women. Both men and women struggle to lose weight due to hormonal changes, metabolism slowing down, and other factors. That is why it's important to seek the guidance of a professional who can provide you with personalized advice and support.

One type of professional to consider seeking help from is a therapist or counselor. Weight loss can be an emotional journey, and it is important to address any underlying issues that may be contributing to your struggles. A therapist can help you uncover and work through any emotional barriers that are holding you back from reaching your goals. They can also provide you with coping strategies and support to help you stay on track.

Overall, seeking professional help on your weight loss journey can increase your chances of success. Whether it is working with a nutritionist, personal trainer, therapist, or all the above, these professionals can provide you with the tools, support, and guidance you need to achieve your weight loss goals. Do not be afraid to reach out and ask for help – you deserve to feel slim, strong, and confident at any age.

Building a Support System

Building a support system is essential when embarking on a weight loss journey. It can be challenging to make lifestyle changes on your own, and having a support system in place can make all the difference. Whether it is friends, family, or a weight loss group, having people to lean on for encouragement and accountability can help you stay motivated and on track toward your goals. One way to build a support system is to enlist the help of a workout friend. Having someone to exercise with can make workouts more. enjoyable and help you stay committed to your fitness routine. It can also provide a sense of camaraderie and encouragement, as you work towards your weight loss goals together.

Herbal Supplements

Herbs can play a supportive role in weight loss by:

- **Enhancing Metabolism**: Herbs like green tea extract and cayenne pepper contain compounds that can boost metabolism and promote fat burning.
- **Suppressing Appetite**: Fenugreek and glucomannan (from konjac root) are known to help reduce appetite and control hunger by increasing feelings of fullness.

- **Balancing Blood Sugar**: Cinnamon and chromium can help stabilize blood sugar levels, which may reduce cravings and prevent insulin spikes.

3. Support for Digestive Health

4. Optimal digestive function is crucial for weight management.

- **Probiotics**: To support a healthy gut microbiome, which can influence weight regulation and appetite control.
- **Detoxification**: Herbal detoxifiers like milk thistle and dandelion root may support liver function and help the body eliminate excess waste
- **Digestive Enzymes**- improve nutrient absorption and reduce bloating.

CHAPTER 12:
Identifying and Overcoming Plateaus

Plateaus are a common occurrence in any weight loss journey, but they can be particularly frustrating for people who like to weigh themselves every day. It is important to understand what causes plateaus and how to overcome them to continue making progress toward your weight loss goals.

Think of plateaus this way. It is a signal from your body that it is bored with what you are doing with nutrition and exercise and means that you need to switch things up to "shock" your body guessing. Plateaus are frustrating for all of us, but they are normal and necessary to help the body change and adapt as you lose weight. There are things that you can do to prolong and, in some cases, completely avoid plateaus.

How To Avoid Plateaus

A lack of variety in your exercise routine ensures that your body will become accustomed to the same workouts, leading to a decrease in the effectiveness of your efforts. It is important to switch up your routine regularly to keep your body challenged and continuously burning calories. Many women like the idea of being consistent with their eating plan and prefer to eat the same meals every day. This is one of the top reasons why the body will stall. Just like exercise workouts you need to switch up your meals each week. Another factor that can contribute to plateaus is not

tracking your food intake accurately. It is easy to underestimate the number of calories you're consuming, which can hinder your weight loss progress. Keeping a food journal and being mindful of portion sizes can help you stay on track and avoid hitting a plateau.

Stress and lack of sleep can also play a role in your weight loss efforts. When you are under stress, your body releases cortisol, a hormone that can lead to weight gain and make it harder to lose weight. Prioritizing self-care practices such as meditation, yoga, and getting enough sleep can help you manage stress and break through plateaus.

Over-exercising and restricting your calories too much can hinder your progress and cause your body to hold onto weight. Taking a week to rest and focusing on nourishing your body with healthy foods can help reset your metabolism and jumpstart your weight loss once again. By identifying the causes of plateaus and making necessary adjustments, you can successfully navigate through them and continue your journey to become slim and strong.

CHECKPOINT TIP: Ask yourself- Am I really at a plateau or have I been eating too many calories and just maintaining weight? Or have I been cutting back on calories too much and my body is holding on to the weight?

How to Break Through a Plateau

Fasting is quite common these days. If you have a lot of weight to lose- long-term fasting is not the answer. You will lose muscle and loose skin when you do reach your goal weight. Short cycles sprinkled throughout your weight loss journey will move you toward your goal faster.

Cheat Meals – Should You Have Them?

Cheating meals are an important part of achieving lifelong weight management. The key is to plan them in and make them 100% worth it. It is not healthy for any of us to completely restrict ourselves from things that we enjoy. Here are a few tips on how to incorporate cheat meals into your weight loss plan.

Step 1. Decide what the cheat meal will be. What is the type of cheat meal that you want to have? Is it a dessert, an alcoholic drink, or a decadent meal with a lot of carbs? Plan it in your meal plan. If it is a dessert cheat meal – eat some protein before you start eating the dessert (chicken or string cheese). Protein is very satiating and will help you to not overeat the dessert.

Step 2. What time of day are you going to be having the meal? If it is a dinner cheat meal, then plan to eat lightly on that day. Protein breakfast, protein meal, or protein snack for lunch then have your dinner as the cheat meal. Get right back on track the next day with your nutrition plan.

Step 3. Think before you eat the cheat meal. Is it something that you will enjoy, or do you just want it because you are bored with your regular weight loss eating plan? If so, find a healthy recipe swap for the cheat meal. Example: If it is a Taco Bell then find a recipe that looks similar and make that instead. Get right back on your plan at the next meal or snack time and add an extra workout in the next day or two to burn off extra calories.

Step 4. Additional thoughts to consider on cheating meals. Sometimes cheat meals can trigger people back into old eating habits and they lose focus on their weight loss goals. It is fine to have cheat meals once a week if you are far enough along on your weight loss journey and you feel ready to manage it and avoid overdoing it or binging.

TIP: I recommend my clients wait at least 6 weeks before adding in cheat meals. They also must have been losing steadily for the 6 weeks.

TIP 2: If there is a specific food that you constantly keep thinking about or that you are obsessed with- **either have the cheat meal** and move on or have a similar swap, eat it, and get back on track.

You should also be cautious about adding cheat meals if you are struggling with emotional eating or binges. In this case, I would prolong them as much as you can so that you can lose a good amount of weight before testing yourself with more tempting foods.

Emotional Eating- Triggers and Social Events

Emotional eating is a frequent problem for many and can be THE catalyst that slows or stops weight loss. A common scenario that you may be dealing with is when you have a great day of staying on track with meals, and then one episode (or binge) of eating a lot of food sets you back an entire week because of the extra calories.

TIP: Think before you eat. Wait 5 full minutes and drink a glass of water before you take a bite. Ask yourself. "Will I regret eating this on the other side?" Are you eating your feelings in this moment?

The emotional aspect of eating cannot be overlooked, especially as women face various life changes. Feelings of nostalgia can be triggered by certain foods, reminding individuals of cherished memories or comforting times. Stress and anxiety can lead to cravings for high-sugar, high-fat foods as a form of self-soothing. Recognizing the emotions that drive these cravings is a critical step in breaking the cycle of emotional eating. By identifying triggers—whether they be social situations, special people, or stressors- you can develop healthier strategies for coping with emotions without turning to food as a solution.

TIP: If you are struggling with anxiety and use food to help "soothe or Stuff" your feelings, the root cause of this could be an unhealthy gut or "leaky gut" because there is a gut and brain connection.

The gut/brain connection. If you have an unhealthy gut, it is feeding the anxiety. I see this a lot in my practice, and it is becoming more and more common. Seek out a healthcare provider who understands leaky gut. As I previously mentioned, conventional medicine doctors typically do not address it as a health condition but in the natural health world, it is a very REAL problem.

Have you ever noticed how most social events and interactions often revolve around food? This can create complex dynamics for people trying to lose weight. You may feel compelled to indulge in foods you might otherwise avoid due to the influence of friends, family, or cultural norms. Recognizing that it's acceptable to set boundaries is the first step in reclaiming personal agency over dietary choices. This can start with simple affirmations such as expressing preferences for certain types of food or declining offerings politely. By communicating these boundaries clearly, you can help create an environment that respects your choices while also encouraging others to consider their eating habits.

You can be successful with weight loss even if you have an active social life. It is more challenging, but it just requires a little strategic planning and will become second nature the more you do it. When you are attending social events, stay strong in what is best for you. It is also important to identify all the emotional triggers that accompany social eating. For many, food serves as a source of comfort or a way to bond with others. However, this can lead to emotional eating, where the act of consuming food becomes a response to stress, loneliness, or anxiety.

Some people may find themselves in situations where they feel pressured to conform to group norms, leading to overeating or unhealthy choices. By recognizing these triggers, you can develop alternative coping strategies, such as engaging in conversation or participating in activities that do not center around food, thereby reducing the likelihood of emotional eating.

Tip: Don't allow others to set you back or delay progress on your weight loss journey. Excel calories and insulin spike delay progress. Before you indulge in something you don't care about, think about how you will feel after eating it. Will you regret it?

TIP 2: Before indulging in an emotional eating event, ask yourself, "Is Is this food worth doing another workout this week to burn off the

I will consume hundreds of extra calories. If the answer is no, then either leave the event or use that to check in with yourself to avoid eating the food.

Peer pressure also plays a considerable role in social situations, often subtly influencing food choices. Friends or family members may encourage indulgence, whether through comments about "just one more bite" or by presenting food as a reward for social engagement. This pressure can be particularly potent among women who have historically prioritized the needs and preferences of others over their own. Learning to assert personal boundaries when it comes to food choices is VITAL in counteracting this influence and promoting a healthier self-image.

Being mindful of these environmental triggers and developing strategies to navigate them —such as choosing smaller portions, alternating alcoholic beverages with water, or planning—can empower women to reclaim control over their food choices during social gatherings. Understanding and addressing these common triggers can be pivotal in preventing emotional eating and fostering a more positive relationship with food in social contexts.

TIP: If you are feeling pressured at an event to have an alcoholic drink or food- take a small portion, have a bite, and pretend to eat it. The point is "How will they know how much you are eating?" They won't know, they just want to see that you are taking it. Do what you need to do to stay in control of the situation, so you do not have regrets later.

Challenging Friendships & Weight Loss

Unfortunately, when it comes to weight loss, women can be very tough on each other. This is because weight loss is a very personal and emotional process. It makes us feel vulnerable and each woman deals with it in her way. So, you either have a group of women who are supportive or are on the same type of journey as you, or, you have some obstacles that you must face regarding handling your friends. It is common for one friend in the group to unexpectedly feel jealous when close friends are successful at weight loss. Most women battle with weight at some point and when someone looks as though they are successful it may cause your friends to face some body image issues of their own. Perhaps they feel like a failure–or think you'll see them as one–because of their unsuccessful weight loss attempts. I have seen this scenario hundreds of times and the main thing to remember is that you are on an important journey and don't let anyone delay or stop your success.

Another reason women struggle with each other's weight loss success is envy. They want what you have. People are most likely to feel jealous over something they think is very important in life. If your friend values thinness and you now weigh less than they do, it could trigger jealousy.

Be patient with your friends but stand your ground and only choose the food that will help you move closer to your goal.

Family members and Food Pushers

Family members, just like friends, can either be supportive or they can be difficult to handle. Especially at holidays when food is the main event.

TIP: The same guidelines apply to family members. Explain your journey if that helps and do what is best for you. Otherwise, it is time to develop the skill of pretending and "finessing your way through the meals.

How Does Alcohol Affect Weight Loss

A good way to approach alcohol if you are trying to lose weight as though it is a cheating meal. Alcohol often leads to cravings for foods that will increase your blood sugar quickly like low-fiber starches. The dehydration and electrolyte imbalance also caused by drinking increases cravings for salty foods like French fries or chips. Have you ever noticed that you want something salty after a night of drinking? And, of course, the more food you consume the more calories there are for your body to work through before getting back to fat-burning

Alcohol can make or break your weight loss each week. Incorporating alcohol strategically will help you stay on track with your weight loss goals. All alcohol is immediately digested into the body as sugar. Understanding how alcohol impacts your weight loss and choosing to have alcohol when it is important, such as on a special occasion is the secret.

How To Incorporate Alcohol & Maximize Weight Loss

<u>Alcohol or Tequila.</u> Have a shot or something diet (juice seltzer) Or a skinny margarita

<u>Red</u> wine is the best but red and white wine are sugar. Yes, red wine does have some excellent health benefits but if you are not yet at your maintenance goal then you need to plan it strategically."

<u>Beer</u>- When you drink beer (any kind) it will slow down weight loss for 48 hours because it is yeast and sugar. If you are eating a meal with beer, it will double the potential for that entire meal to be stored as fat.

Tip 4: Plan an extra workout (the next day) after drinking alcohol to minimize the impact on your metabolism. As alcohol wreaks havoc with your metabolism, it launches a second assault to sabotage weight loss. The more you drink, the more your brain and body desire more food.

It is always ok to choose to have alcohol when you feel it is important. The key is to understand how it may affect your goals and make the best possible choice.

Quick reference – Incorporating Alcohol

1). Choose wine or hard liquor over beer. Beer is all yeast and sugar.

2) Tequilla or vodka shots (or with seltzer) will be the best choice to minimize the impact of alcohol on slowing down the metabolism.

2) Don't drink and eat at the same time. Wait at least 30 minutes before eating if possible.

3) Plan and incorporate the alcohol into your day- do not drink spontaneously!

4) Plan to exercise the day after having alcohol.

5) Make it 100% worth it.

Many of my clients have found that if they prioritize each social event and plan for alcohol, it helps them to stay in control and they avoid feeling that they are missing out. You do not have to completely avoid alcohol while you are trying to lose weight. If you decide to have it, enjoy it. Have a plan in place to offset the extra calories and minimize the impact on your blood sugar levels. Avoid drinking alcohol with carbs, highly processed foods, and sugary drinks as much as possible, because they can contribute to weight gain and other health issues. It is ok to enjoy a glass of wine from time to time. The goal is to minimize alcohol as much as possible until you are close to your goal but add it back in slowly as you approach the last 5 pounds of your weight loss goal.

Welcome to Maintenance

I define maintenance as achieving a weight that feels good internally and physically. Maintenance means) sugar management does not mean you stay at the same number on the scale. Maintenance is a "range" of numbers. For example, if you feel good at 145, your maintenance range is 144 – 147. You always want to consider the "fluid factor." This means your body will always fluctuate in terms of water weight. If you don't feel your sweet spot weight is 147, move your range down to 142- 145. Lose a few more pounds then adjust your maintenance range.

When you reach your weight loss goal this means you have successfully mastered the obstacles that typically caused your weight gain. Congratulations! Think of all the obstacles you have tackled along the way. Social eating, temptations, emotional eating, meal planning, exercise routine, and your personalized nutrition plan and, hopefully, you are on your way to healing the root causes that caused you to have excess weight in the first place.

What is Your Maintenance Range

Maintenance Range- This means that you are up 3 or down three on the scale. from your goal weight. This is the range in which you "live." and monitor your weight.

TIP: If you are doing well staying in your maintenance range but you feel like your belly is starting to feel "thick" or distended again, then you have been eating things that are elevating your blood sugar too much. Look back at your journals or start tracking where and what sources the excess sugar is coming from and make the appropriate adjustments asap.

Consistency- Sustainable weight loss is focusing on what you have learned so far about your body. What does it respond well to? What healthy foods make you feel good? Has your exercise routine felt good so far and can you sustain it for the next few months? Or 6 months?

How is your family and work life since reaching your goal? Do you feel the healthy lifestyle transition is going well and will be sustainable? If not, jot down the things that need attention and plan to address them.

Understanding your individual carbohydrate tolerance is vital for effective meal planning. Each person's body reacts differently to carbohydrates based on factors like genetics, activity level, and health conditions. Keeping a food diary or utilizing apps that track carbohydrate intake can help individuals identify how different foods affect their energy levels and overall well-being. By tailoring carbohydrate consumption to personal needs and preferences, those over 40 can create meal strategies that promote energy, support weight management, and enhance overall health.

A carb threshold refers to the maximum amount of carbohydrates that an individual can consume without adversely affecting their weight, blood sugar levels, or overall health. This threshold varies from person to person, influenced by factors such as age, activity level, metabolic rate, and personal health conditions. Recognizing where your carb threshold lies can empower you to make informed dietary choices and optimize your meal planning. The question becomes – how many carbs can I eat and maintain my weight?

Your body's ability to process carbohydrates may decline due to hormonal changes and slower metabolism, so the key is to test it out. You have learned about the importance of stabilizing blood sugar- and as you enter maintenance. The next step is to identify your threshold, you can tailor your carbohydrate intake to fit your lifestyle, ensuring you consume enough to fuel your body without exceeding the amount that could lead to unwanted health issues. I wish I could give you the exact formula, but it is different, or every

Start with 3 planned meals of carbs in a week, Add a serving into your normal meal 3 to 4 times a week. Continue with your normal exercise routine and see how your body responds that week. Any usual feeling of bloating, cravings coming back fatigued- or did you feel stubby energy? This is how you begin to adapt to enjoying life and eating carbs. Combine to weigh each week on the 7th day- and based on your result make the appropriate adjustment. I have found that most people's plans can comfortably have 3- 5 meals and maintain their weight.

To determine your carb threshold, start by tracking your daily carbohydrate intake along with any physical and emotional responses you experience. Pay attention to how your body reacts after meals: Do you feel energized or sluggish? Do you experience cravings or mood swings? Keeping a food diary can help you identify patterns and adjust as necessary. Additionally, consulting with a healthcare professional or a nutritionist can provide valuable insights tailored to your specific needs. They can help you establish a balanced meal plan that respects your carb threshold while ensuring you receive the necessary nutrients.

Meal planning becomes a vital tool in managing your carb threshold effectively. By preparing meals in advance, you can control portion sizes and choose the right types of carbohydrates, such as whole grains, fruits, and vegetables, which offer fiber and nutrients without causing significant spikes in blood sugar.

Planning also allows you to incorporate a variety of foods, helping you avoid the monotony that can lead to cravings or overeating. By sticking to a structured meal plan, you can maintain your carb intake within your desired threshold while enjoying a diverse and satisfying diet.

Ultimately, understanding your carb threshold is about more than just numbers; it's about fostering a healthier relationship with food. As you navigate through meal planning over the next few months and beyond, aim to prioritize whole nutrient-dense foods while being mindful of your carbohydrate consumption. By doing so, you can enjoy the benefits of stable energy levels, improved mood, and long-term health. Embracing carb control as part of your lifestyle will contribute significantly to your overall well-being, making it easier to maintain your health and vitality as you age.

Final Tips and Reminders on Maintenance:

- Pay attention to how your clothes fit.
- Cheat meal- enjoy but plan.

- Plam your week based on your social events.
- Tune in and listen to your body signals. Trust them.
- Plan for social events and incorporate alcohol wisely.
- Always have grab-and-go snacks with you.
- Plan your carbs each week. Know your carb threshold.
- Develop sustainable habits.
- Batch Cook as often as possible.

From a naturopathic standpoint, sustaining weight loss goes beyond mere caloric restriction and instead emphasizes a holistic approach to overall well-being. I want to encourage you to explore the world of naturopathy to help you during the next chapter in your life. It will help bring awareness to harmonizing the body's natural rhythms and promoting balance through your new lifestyle adjustments. As you continue to integrate diet rich as a whole, unprocessed foods that support your unique metabolic health. such as fresh vegetables, fruits, nuts, and lean proteins.

I hope this book helped you feel more confident that you can lose and maintain your weight loss and feel equipped to tackle the obstacles that have kept you from losing weight. If you do not have a trusted healthcare provider or nutritional therapist who can help you reach your goals, please reach out to me via my website DrLoriMahler.com, or contact me directly at Drlorimahler@gmail.com. and schedule a virtual consultation.

I would like to leave you with some of my healthy dessert recipes to incorporate into your maintenance plan.

10 Healthy desserts .pdf - My patients' top picks!

Thanks so much for taking the time to read my book. If you enjoyed it, please leave a review so that I can help as many people as I can reach their weight loss goals.

Stay on Track with Your
Maintenance
Goal

10 Healthy Desserts

Best of health to you and your family!

Dr. Lori Mahler